Ethnicity and Nursing Practice

Edited by

Lorraine Culley and Simon Dyson

palgrave

First published 2001 by
PALGRAVE
Houndmills, Basingstoke, Hampshire RG21 6XS and
175 Fifth Avenue, New York, N.Y. 10010
Companies and representatives throughout the world

PALGRAVE is the new global academic imprint of
St. Martin's Press LLC Scholarly and Reference Division and
Palgrave Publishers Ltd (formerly Macmillan Press Ltd).

ISBN 0–333–75331–3

This book is printed on paper suitable for recycling and made from fully managed and sustained forest sources.

A catalogue record for this book is available from the British Library.

10   9   8   7   6   5   4   3   2   1
10   09   08   07   06   05   04   03   02   01

Printed in Malaysia

60361809 X

In memory of May Culley (1920–2000)
and
for Rehana and Ingrid

Contents

List of tables

Series editors' preface

It is widely accepted that because sociology can provide nurses with valuable and pertinent insights, it should be a constituent part of nursing's knowledge base. To take but a few substantive examples, sociology can help nurses understand the causes and distribution of ill health, the experience of illness, the dynamics of health care encounters and the limitations and possibilities of professional care. Equally important, sociology's emphasis on critical reflection can encourage nurses to be more questioning and self-aware, thus helping them to provide flexible, non discriminatory, client-centred care.

Unfortunately, while the aspiration of integrating sociology into nursing knowledge is easy enough to state in theory, in practice their relationship has not been as productive as some might have hoped. Notwithstanding several works which have successfully applied sociological tools to nursing problems, there remains a gulf between the two disciplines which has led some to question the utility of the relationship.

On the one hand, sociologists, while taking an interest in nursing's occupational position, have not paid great attention to the actual work that nurses do. This is partially due to the limitations of sociological surveillance. Nurses work in confidential, private and intimate settings with their clients. Sociologists' access to such settings is necessarily restricted. Moreover, nurses find it difficult to talk about their work, except to other nurses. As a result, core issues pertaining to nursing have been less than thoroughly treated in the sociological literature. There is thus a disjunction between what nurses require from sociology and what sociologists can provide.

On the other hand, nurses are on equally uncertain ground when they attempt to use sociology themselves. Often nurses are reliant on carefully simplified introductory texts which, because of their broad remit, are often unable to provide in-depth understanding of sociological insights. Nor is it simply a matter of knowledge; there are tensions between the outlooks of nursing and sociology. Because nursing work involves individual interactions, it is not surprising that when nurses turn to sociology, they turn to those elements which concentrate on micro-social interaction. While it is useful in so far as it goes, it does not provide nurses with knowledge of the restraints and enablements imposed upon individual actions by social structures.

The aim of the *Sociology and Nursing Practice* series is to bridge these gaps between the disciplines. The authors of the series are nurses or teachers of nurses and therefore have an intimate understanding of nursing work and an appreciation of the importance of individualized nursing care. Yet at the same time, they are committed to a sociological outlook that asserts the salience of wider social forces to the work of nurses. The texts apply sociological theories and concepts to practical aspects of nursing. They explore nursing care as part of the social world, showing how different approaches to understanding the relationship between the individual and society have implications for nursing practice. By concentrating on specific aspects of sociology or nursing, each book is able to provide the reader with a deeper knowledge of those aspects of sociology most pertinent to their own area of work or study. We hope the series will encourage nurses to analyse critically their practice and profession and to develop their own contribution to health care.

Margaret Miers, Sam Porter and Geoff Wilkinson

Acknowledgements

The publishers and the editors would like to thank the following for permission to publish copyright material:

The Office for National Statistics for permission to reproduce the material in Tables 2.1; 2.2; 2.4; and Table 4.1;

The Head of Publications, Policy Studies Institute, London for permission to reproduce material in Table 2.5 and Table 9.1;

Crown copyright material is reproduced with permission of the Controller of Her Majesty's Stationery Office (Table 2.3);

The Health Development Agency for permission to use the data that comprise Table 7.1.

We would like to thank the Series Editors for their support and encouragement, especially Sam Porter for constructive suggestions throughout. Thanks are also due to all the contributors for speedy responses to editorial suggestions. We would also like to thank Anne Clarke for her help in checking references and indexing the book.

Lorraine would like to thank Jack Demaine for his encouragement, Tom and Will for the time stolen from them to complete the book.

Simon would also like to thank all his family and friends who have helped care for Rehana and Ingrid to enable him to go to work at all, including Wendy and Rachel Young, Garry Bond, Jean and Peter Dyson, Melanie and Tony Vieira, Tony Lawson, Anne and Phil Brown, Nicky and Mike Drucquer, Clive and Chrissie Gray, Alistair and Claire Jones, Dave and Elaine Hiles, and Yvette, Paula and Grace Taylor.

Lorraine Culley and Simon Dyson

Notes on contributors

Hannah Bradby studied and worked in the Medical Research Council Medical Sociology Unit in Glasgow for nine years before moving to a lectureship at the University of Warwick's Department of Sociology. She speaks fluent French, elementary Hindi, minimal Punjabi and tourist Italian.

Mel Chevannes CBE FRCN is Professor of Nursing, Head of School of Nursing and Midwifery, and Director of the Mary Seacole Research Centre at De Montfort University, Leicester. Her research focuses on child rearing among the black Caribbean community in Britain, community care for older people, and the contribution of nurses to a multi ethnic society.

Lorraine Culley is a Reader in Health Studies in the Faculty of Health and Community Studies at De Montfort University, Leicester. Her current research interests include ethnicity and health, the experiences of minority ethnic workers, equal opportunities, and infertility and health policy.

Simon Dyson is a Principal Lecturer in Health Studies in the Faculty of Health and Community Studies at De Montfort University, Leicester. He is the author of *Mental Handicap: Dilemmas of Parent-Professional Relations* (Croom Helm, 1987) and is currently researching social aspects of sickle cell/thalassaemia.

Yasmin Gunaratnam is a Research Fellow in the School of Health and Social Welfare at the Open University. Her interest in issues of 'race', ethnicity and palliative care arose out of her experiences as a carer for her mother during a terminal illness. She explored these issues further in her PhD at the London School of Economics. She lives in London and has a two-year-old son.

Silvia Ham-Ying is a Principal Lecturer in Nursing in the Faculty of Health and Community Studies at De Montfort

University, Leicester. Her current research interests include holistic health care, transcultural nursing and continuing professional development.

Karen Iley is a Senior Lecturer in Sociology at the Faculty of Health, Southbank University, London. Her teaching interests include health inequalities, ethnicity and gender. She is also an experienced registered nurse who has worked as practitioner and manager in several acute care settings in culturally diverse inner city hospitals.

Mark R D Johnson is Reader in Primary Care, and Associate Director of the Mary Seacole Research Centre, De Montfort University, Leicester. He has published widely about multi-agency health and welfare service delivery sensitive to ethnic and cultural diversity, barriers to access, and appropriate research methods to investigate these issues.

Vina Mayor is Head of Department – Community and Primary Care Nursing at City University, London. Her research interests are ethnicity and health, nursing careers, especially those of ethnic minority nurses and primary care practice development. She is nearing the completion of her PhD studies focusing on the careers of leading black nurses in England.

Jon Mulholland is a Lecturer in Sociology at the Wolfson Institute of Health and Human Sciences, Thames Valley University, where he is the module leader for 'Ethnicity, Culture and Health' and 'Social Psychology and Health'. He is currently completing a PhD addressing the themes of racialization and sexual science.

James Nazroo is Senior Lecturer in Sociology in the Department of Epidemiology and Public Health, University College London. Ethnic inequalities in health and mental health have been a major focus of his research activities. This has involved both describing differences across groups and assessing the contribution that social disadvantage might make to these.

Chris Smaje is a Lecturer in Sociology at the University of Surrey. He has written and researched extensively on the health and health care of minority ethnic groups, and also on the sociology of race and ethnicity. He is the author of *Health, Race* *and Ethnicity: Making Sense of the Evidence* (King's Fund, 1995) and *Natural Hierarchies: The Historical Sociology of Race and Caste* (Blackwell, 2000).

Wendy Young was formerly a Research Assistant in the Department of Health and Continuing Professional Studies at De Montfort University, Leicester.

Introduction: sociology, ethnicity and nursing practice

Lorraine Culley and Simon Dyson

There is a growing body of evidence to suggest that Britain's health services are not adequately meeting the needs of minority ethnic groups. This failure occurs across many settings and takes many forms (Ahmad 1993, 2000; Culley 2000). The nursing profession has also been specifically challenged in this respect (Thomas and Dines 1994; Rudat 1994; Douglas 1995) and recent research has been quite critical of the educational preparation of nurses for professional practice in a multi-ethnic society (Gerrish *et al.* 1996). This book aims to assist the nursing profession's clear desire to ensure that nurses are equipped with the necessary competencies to meet the health care needs of minority ethnic communities by offering perspectives and insights from sociological theory and empirical research.

Ethnicity and Nursing Practice aims to provide an outline of sociological concepts relating to 'race' and ethnicity and a demonstration of the relevance of these concepts to nursing practice. It is hoped that it will help nurses to appreciate the broader context of nursing practice and the social and political significance of ethnicity in contemporary Britain. The book aims to do this in a way which is somewhat different from the perhaps more familiar perspective of transcultural nursing. Within the professional discourse of nursing, the issue of 'race' and ethnicity is dominated by an essentialist concept of culture, heavily influenced by Leininger's pioneering work on transcultural nursing (Leininger 1991). The contributors to *Ethnicity and Nursing Practice* reflect the perspective that, while it is important to respond to cultural diversity in professional practice, adherence to an essentialist view of culture has serious drawbacks. Although the book is a collection of discrete chapters addressing specific issues of theory or practice, there are several themes which run through these contributions and which signal a need to rethink some current perspectives on ethnicity and nursing.

One central theme of the book relates to the concept of ethnicity. As indicated above, the contributors are critical of the idea of ethnicity as a fixed and static set of cultural attributes. There are many who now criticize a concept of ethnicity based on the idea that there is a stable set of cultural traits or attributes which people 'possess' and which define them. This is what has been called an essentialist concept of ethnicity and it can easily lead to harmful stereotyping. Those who criticize this view of ethnicity propose an alternative view of ethnicity as more malleable, as fluid and mutable. Ethnic identities are subject to change and redefinition and cannot therefore be easily captured in a cultural checklist. The idea of 'situational ethnicity', discussed in several chapters of the book, suggests that different aspects of a patient's ethnic identification may become relatively more or relatively less important in any given context. So for example, it is possible to be 'simultaneously English, British and European, stressing these identities more or less strongly in different aspects of daily life. Similarly the same person might identify as Gujarati, Indian, Hindu, East African Asian or British depending on situation, immediate objectives, and the responses and behaviour of others' (Mason 1995: 13). This is discussed in more detail in Chapter 1, and in Chapters 5 and 8, where it is argued that an essentialist perspective can give rise to professional anxieties and stifle good practice. Cultural and religious needs are negotiable. Nurses need to use communication skills to ascertain rather than assume what preferences and practices are of significance to users.

A second and related theme of the book is the importance of recognizing and responding to diversity. There is considerable diversity *between* groups commonly defined as minority ethnic groups. This diversity of experience extends to all aspects of life, including education, housing, employment, and indeed health (Modood *et al.* 1997). As recent research has highlighted, it makes very little sense to talk in general terms about 'the health of ethnic minorities' (Nazroo 1997a). There is considerable diversity in the health status and possibly also the health care of different minority ethnic groups, although the latter is under-researched.

There is, of course, also considerable diversity *within* groups defined as 'ethnic groups'. Ethnic groups are not homogenous. They are divided by class, gender, generation and sexual orientation, as well as by a range of other statuses that might be relevant in specific contexts. One should of course, add to this the diversity of individual attributes such as personality. There is a tendency to define members of minority ethnic groups solely in terms of their ethnicity in a way which is not applied to the ethnic majority. To refer to a patient as 'Asian' or even 'Indian' tells us little that could be of use in providing appropriate health care, any more than would referring to a patient as 'white'.

The third major theme of the book concerns the need for health professionals to have an awareness of the socio-political context of a multiethnic society. It is vital for nurses to be aware of the historical context which frames the current ethnic patterning of Britain. It is also important that nurses are alert to the realities of racism which affect all minority ethnic groups and the forms of social and economic disadvantage which impact upon both the health status and the health care of most minority ethnic groups. Some of the historical background to migration is discussed in Chapter 11, and references to the socio-economic context occur throughout the book. There are, in addition, many accounts of ethnic inequalities in housing, education, employment, social services and the criminal justice system to which nurses could usefully refer (Mason 1995; Modood *et al.* 1997). Discussions of racism, racial abuse and racial violence as significant aspects of the experience of many members of minority ethnic groups are also highly relevant to an understanding of health and healthcare (Virdee 1995).

Our experience as sociologists involved in nurse education indicates that there is a great deal to be done in clarifying concepts of 'race', ethnicity and ethnic identities as a crucial starting point for any discussion of nursing practice and this will be reflected in the content of several chapters of the book. For the moment however, this introductory chapter will briefly discuss a number of terminological issues which we hope will assist the reader to become aware of the origins or the implications of certain concepts which may work against the provision of appropriate nursing practice. It will then go on to outline the structure of the book.

'Race', racism and ethnicity: terminology and concepts

Discussions of 'race', racism and ethnicity are particularly difficult for students who are relatively new to social science, since there are many competing terms and concepts employed to describe and analyse these phenomena. To some extent this mirrors the situation in popular and in political and administrative contexts, where the terms 'race' and ethnicity are frequently used interchangeably, sometimes even in the same sentence (Fenton 1999). While it is not possible to review this issue in any depth here (but see Mason 1995 and Fenton 1999, as well as Mulholland and Dyson in this volume) it is important to briefly introduce some key notes of caution with respect to terminology.

As we shall see in Chapter 1, the notion that there are groups of people so biologically distinct that they form separate racial groups or races has been scientifically discredited. There is a great deal of genetic variation within the so-called 'races' and a great deal of genetic overlap between them. Therefore terms such as 'Caucasian', which are part of such a scheme of racial classification, are inappropriate since they carry clear connotations of biological race. It is also important to remember that the idea of biological races has also been associated historically with much malevolence and hatred. The initial misguided classification of people into separate 'races' took place at a time when Britain had a colonial empire and the classification was based on the notion of a hierarchy of 'races' (i.e. some 'races' were allegedly superior to others).

Some sociologists argue against using the term race at all, preferring the term ethnicity to refer to *socially constructed* differences, grounded in culture, ancestry and language rather than in supposed physical or biological differences. Others have argued that the term 'race' should be maintained but use the term in inverted commas ('race') to signal that they are using the word in the social rather than the biological sense. One argument here is that while race has no scientific basis, many people still think and act as if there really were distinct racial groups and therefore notions of racial difference continue to be highly influential.

A further example of the difficulty of terminology is provided by the use of the term 'black'. This is commonly used in discussions of 'race' and health. However, even in published research studies, all too often such terms are not clearly defined and we read accounts of 'black and minority ethnic groups', or 'black groups' without any clear understanding of the collectivities being referred to (Sheldon and Parker 1992). Sometimes 'black' is used to refer to all minority ethnic groups and sometimes it refers only to African and African-Caribbean groups. This can lead to confusing and potentially misleading accounts.

The term 'black' was adopted by those keen to stress the commonalities in the experience of oppression of all minority ethnic groups by a dominant white racism and concerned to present a political opposition to it (Mason 1995) and in the 1970s and '80s the term acquired a considerable popular usage. The proposition here was that as racists represent all non-white people as 'black' this is the appropriate sociological description for all such groups (Modood *et al.* 1994). More recently however, the use of this term has been challenged on several grounds. While 'black' has perhaps been the predominant term of self-identity among many Caribbeans, some sociologists have argued that people from the Indian subcontinent do not readily define themselves as 'black' (Modood 1998). It is also suggested that a further problem concerns the way in which this view sets up a 'black–white' opposition. That is, there is a tendency to assume that society can be neatly divided into an oppressed black minority and a dominant white majority. Such an opposition, however, is regarded by many as oversimplistic. It has the effect of polarizing groups, ignoring differences such as gender and class, within both 'black' and 'white' groups and it encourages the view of ethnic minorities as passive victims of racism. Such a view also suggests an oversimplified and inaccurate view of racism as confined to a black–white opposition. Those who are keen to stress the diversity of cultural differences argue that the use of the term 'black', while sometimes a useful shorthand, masks the very real differences of identity, history and tradition which are important in how people define themselves.

The term 'white' is also used in a confusing and ambiguous manner, often employed interchangeably with English or British or European. This confuses notions of nationality or citizenship with concepts of ethnicity. It is far from clear that the term 'white' has any clear or unambiguous meaning. As we shall argue in Chapter 5, the concept 'white' needs to be subjected to some long overdue scrutiny. In the context of health differences, it is clear that there are 'white' minority groups such as the Irish, whose needs are often overlooked.

As a reflection of the ambiguity and the political nature of terminology in this area, many nurses may feel uncertain about the use of language and may fear offending clients. As a result, some may try to find words that 'feel' less stark than, say, the term black. One such word is 'coloured'. But we need to be aware that under the twentieth century racist regime of apartheid in South Africa, the term 'coloured' became part of a classification of 'races' used by the state in effecting systematic discrimination. To this extent the term 'coloured' is therefore potentially offensive to many people. Another common term is 'immigrant', which is frequently used inappropriately to refer to all members of minority ethnic groups. While this might be an accurate description of many elders in minority ethnic groups, the majority of members of minority ethnic groups are born in the UK. In addition, the majority of migrants to this country are white. It is also important to recognise that 'immigrant' is a highly political and controversial term and has been used in media reporting and in political speeches over the past 50 years as a pejorative term to promote fear and tension between communities (see Silverman 1993: 79).

As we have seen, some sociologists have argued that the term ethnicity is more appealing than the problematic concept of race. However, the problem of terminology also extends to the idea of ethnicity. There is no single, universally accepted concept of ethnicity and this book is concerned with challenging some of the ideas about ethnicity which predominate in nursing. Ethnicity is socially constructed and socially grounded in culture, ancestry and language (Fenton 1999). Ethnicity is generally used in sociology to refer to peoples with a common ancestry, usually linked to a particular geographical territory, and perhaps sharing a language, religion and other social customs. In nursing texts, however, the complexities of ethnic diversity are often ignored and a potentially damaging view of ethnic groups arises. This is discussed in some detail in Chapters 5 and 8. A variety of approaches to defining ethnicity are discussed in Chapter 1. For the moment it is important to make the point that ethnic identity is concerned with the way in which people define themselves and their relationships to others (Mason 1995).

> Ethnic identity is a product of a number of forces including social exclusion and stigma and political resistance to them, distinctive cultural and religious heritages as well as new forms of culture, communal and familial loyalties, marriage practices, coalition of interests and so on. Hence the boundaries of groups are unclear and shifting. (Modood *et al.* 1994)

There are two further issues relating to terminology which arise in popular discourse and against which nurses need to guard. The first concerns the tendency to confuse ethnicity with nationality. To have British nationality is a specific political and legal status which is conferred on certain citizens of the British State. This is quite distinct from ethnicity, which refers to aspects of cultural distinctiveness much wider than such legal definitions. The second issue concerns the use of the term 'ethnic' to refer to minority ethnic cultures. Nurses may refer to an 'ethnic diet' or to their 'ethnic clients'. However, as the concept of ethnicity outlined above shows, we *all* have ethnicity, we are all ethnic. Most people mark themselves off from others on the basis of some aspect of culture, ancestry or language, although the strength and personal significance of such ethnic identification varies.

Some sociologists have criticized the emphasis on ethnicity because it has appeared to side-step the problem of racism and neglect the inequalities which are evident in racialized societies such as Britain (Fenton 1999). However, although sociologists reject the notion of race, they *are* concerned about *racism*. But in coming to an understanding of the nature and impact of racism there are again difficulties for students new to social science, since racism is what sociologists call a 'contested

concept'. That is, there are strong disagreements over its definition. The term has different meanings in different theoretical
traditions but all too often the term 'racism' is used in an
untheorized and rather sloppy way (Mason 1995). For many
sociologists racism refers to both ideas (attitudes, beliefs and ideologies) and to actions and structures which operate to promote
the exclusion of people by virtue of their being deemed
members of different racial groups (Goldberg 1993). The fact
that such exclusions may take different forms at different times,
leads many to the conclusion that there is no one form of racism,
but rather many *racisms*. The racism that underpinned slavery
in the Caribbean is different in fundamental ways from that
which buttressed British colonial rule in India and from that
which sustains anti-Islamic sentiment in present day Britain.
Particular aspects of racism and racist violence, are illustrated in
the final section of the book.

In examining the impact of racism on health and healthcare,
sociologists are interested in the ways in which different kinds
of racisms may result in some minority ethnic groups (or sections of them) experiencing poverty, high levels of unemployment, hazardous or dangerous employment, poor housing and
educational disadvantage – all of which may impact negatively
on health. They are also interested in whether discriminatory
attitudes of health service staff might lead to some members of
minority ethnic groups facing barriers in accessing services, or
receiving poorer quality care. They are interested in whether
health care providers have policies which can deal with patients
who are racist to other patients. They are interested in the experiences of minority ethnic staff and whether colleagues or
patients act in a discriminatory way towards them. These
sociological concerns are all reflected in the contributions to this
volume in the *Sociology and Nursing Practice* series.

The structure of the book

The book is divided into three broad sections. The first section,
Ethnicity and Health, addresses 'macro' issues in the structuring of 'race', ethnicity and nursing practice. This involves
unpacking the meaning of the concept 'race', describing

ethnicity, identifying racisms, and linking these to inequalities in health statuses and access to services. This section provides a vital conceptual and empirical context to the issue of nursing in a multi-ethnic society.

In the first chapter, Jon Mulholland and Simon Dyson examine some basic issues in thinking about 'race' and ethnicity, including why biological notions of 'race' are not sustainable. It introduces the concept of ethnicity and shows why it is a problem if we think in terms of 'fixed' ethnic groups. The relevance of major social scientific theories to ethnicity and nursing practice is also discussed. Attention is drawn to variations in the extent to which ethnicity is central to the self-identity of patients and the ways in which 'new ethnicities' are dynamically created by patients.

In Chapter 2, Simon Dyson and Chris Smaje discuss the issue of inequalities in health. They note the methodological problems in trying to assess the evidence in this area, the importance of distinguishing death rates and illness rates for particular diseases, and the need to understand when evidence refers to country of birth and when to ethnicity. The chapter outlines patterns of both mortality and morbidity in minority ethnic groups. It also reviews the competing theories that have been offered as a possible explanation of the patterns of minority ethnic health. These include an appraisal of the relative role of genetics in health status; the possible contributions of migration to health status; the direct and indirect effects of racism on health; the issue of access to services; and the contribution of material factors such as poverty; occupation; levels of unemployment; and housing tenure to health status. It offers a critique of simplistic explanations based on culture. However, cultures may in part be forged by material circumstances, while the experience of material circumstances is mediated by culture. In the conclusion nurses are encouraged to distinguish between the underlying causes of inequalities and the manner in which these inequalities are experienced.

Mental illness has been the subject of a number of sociological investigations and in Chapter 3, Karen Iley and James Nazroo look at how rates of mental illness vary both across and within ethnic groups. This discussion demonstrates the importance of taking into account socio-economic factors and shows the ways in which recent research into ethnicity and mental health (Nazroo 1997b) has challenged existing assumptions about the mental health of ethnic minority groups. It provides an opportunity to examine methodological issues in ethnicity and health research and examines evidence relating to the quality of care received by ethnic minority people in mental health care.

Ethnic record keeping and ethnic monitoring are significant issues in the current context of nursing practice and these are considered in Chapter 4. Here, Mark Johnson considers what should be recorded for the purposes of ethnic monitoring and argues that it is appropriate to collect data that are relevant to the particular aspect of service provision under consideration.

The chapter addresses the issue of the purposes of monitoring, its potential drawbacks and criticisms and the differences between the 1991 and 2001 Census categories. Most importantly it examines how ethnic monitoring should be done in practice, considers what guidance exists on implementing monitoring and outlines the training needs of health staff in this area.

The second section of the book *Ethnicity and Practice* focuses on 'micro' issues in the delivery of nursing care. It discusses some of the conceptual and practical difficulties of notions of cultural sensitivity and outlines suggestions for culturally competent and culturally safe nursing. Several specific areas of practice are addressed, including palliative care, midwifery and community health nursing. This section also addresses the more general, but highly relevant, issues of communication and interpretation.

In Chapter 5, Lorraine Culley discusses the debate surrounding the role of culture in understanding differences in health status between ethnic groups. The chapter outlines the potentially damaging consequences for healthcare of an essentialist view of culture. These include a failure to recognize the significance of differences of class, gender, age and other statuses within broadly defined ethnic groups and an overemphasis of difference between ethnic groups. The chapter discusses Ahmad's (1996a) critique of the idea that behaviour is structured according to culturally based health beliefs in a direct and linear way. However, rejecting an essentialist concept of culture does not mean denying that people may draw upon elements of culture to construct ideas about health and responses to illness, although good empirical studies of how this occurs in contemporary Britain are relatively rare. The chapter goes on to identify some of the difficulties of 'transcultural' nursing and suggests limitations to the use of cultural checklists in nursing practice. Alternative ways of approaching cultural competence are suggested and the chapter discusses some of the tensions and dilemmas that nurses might encounter in avoiding practice based on stereotypes.

The lack of bilingual health workers and interpretation services is acknowledged as an ongoing problem in the delivery of healthcare to some members of minority ethnic groups and in Chapter 6, Hannah Bradby considers the issue of communication and interpretation in health care settings. Reliance on relatives or non-clinical minority ethnic staff to interpret breaks confidentiality, risks serious misdiagnosis, and may exacerbate psychological harm. However, effective communication also depends upon nurses being aware of potential variations in meanings at several levels, including the consequences of using colloquial language or professional jargon.

In Chapter 7, Simon Dyson introduces haemoglobin disorders (sickle cell anaemia and beta-thalassaemia) and their prevalence in minority ethnic communities in the UK. Midwifery knowledge of haemoglobin disorders is limited, especially in understanding patterns of inheritance and the particular ethnic groups that may be affected. Confusions in current classificatory practices are outlined. Practical suggestions for effecting selectivity in screening are made. Asking better questions in regard of ethnicity requires better explanations of genetics, a better explanation of the reasons for which information about ethnicity is being sought, and better soliciting of consent for genetic tests. In this way improved understanding of 'race' and ethnicity may be a key to improving many other aspects of the service delivery.

The relative lack of responsiveness of palliative care services to the needs of minority ethnic groups and some possible reasons for this is discussed by Yasmin Gunaratnam in Chapter 8. This failure to adequately address the needs of minority ethnic users of palliative care reflects the wider inadequacies of health

service provision to minority ethnic groups such as lack of interpreters, a lack of facilities to meet diverse religious and cultural
needs and the low numbers of minority ethnic staff. But some
of the problems of providing appropriate palliative care lie
within the so-called multicultural approach to nursing practice.
This approach tends to ignore diversity of experience within
ethnic groups. It fails to take account of how experiences of
racism, sexism and socio-economic factors affects people's experiences of palliative care. And it can prevent nurses from
engaging in the time-consuming work of negotiating choices
about care with the client.

In Chapter 9, Mel Chevannes reviews the issues associated
with working with families from minority ethnic groups. The
chapter examines the inequalities in access to community health
services. Next the changing structures of households are considered, noting the importance of distinguishing between
partnerships, formal marriage, having children, household composition, relationships with kin, and sources of social support.
All of these factors are related in increasingly complex and
changing ways in all ethnic groups. This sociological awareness
is necessary to move beyond crude stereotypes of single-parent
or extended families in working with minority ethnic groups,
and has important implications for community nurse practice.
In the context of wider racism in society, the health check, home
visit, and screening may have different meanings in the context
of the lives of different minority ethnic communities. Resources
are available, but these need to be evaluated rather than merely
picked up and used uncritically. Work-based learning is suggested as a way forward to help the community health nurse
negotiate the care her client is to receive.

The third and final section of the book, *Nurses from Minority Ethnic Groups*, concentrates on the careers of nurses from
minority ethnic groups and looks at how racisms may be experienced and resisted by such groups. It outlines the breadth
of discrimination against minority ethnic nurses, and the limits
of policies designed to address these inequities. It further
describes in depth some responses of minority ethnic nurses to
varied experiences of racism in nursing.

Lorraine Culley and Vina Mayor examine recent evidence
concerning patterns of recruitment of nurses from minority

ethnic groups, their career pathways and experiences of racisms. In Chapter 10, they outline the history of 'overseas' nurses in the National Health Service (NHS) and the current patterns in the ethnic composition of the nursing workforce. They consider recruitment to nurse education and the experiences of minority ethnic student nurses. They also discuss evidence relating to racial discrimination and harassment in nursing and the development and impact of equal opportunities policies. Although there is a long history of policy statements relating to discrimination in the NHS, efforts to tackle this have been piecemeal and fragmented, with very little monitoring of effectiveness. The chapter discusses some of the more recent initiatives designed to develop a workforce representative of a multicultural society.

In the final chapter, together with Silvia Ham-Ying and Wendy Young, we analyse how notions of professionalism interact with the appearance, naming and damaging effects of racism. This draws upon the history of migration from the Caribbean and recruitment of Caribbean nurses to the NHS to examine the interface of racisms and professionalism in nursing. Based on current research using in-depth interviews with 14 Caribbean nurses who came to Britain in the 1950s and '60s, the chapter suggests lessons for developing strategies which acknowledge the complex issues involved in identifying and responding to different forms of racism.

Conclusion

The twentieth century saw many changes in the roles, status and composition of the nursing profession. Nursing history has 're-discovered' the role of the early Caribbean-born nurse pioneer Mary Seacole in developing the art of nursing during the Crimean War. The nursing profession has evolved, especially in the second half of the twentieth century, with the support of nurses of Caribbean, South Asian and Irish descent. At the same time, the ethnic make-up of the client group who are being nursed has become more diverse.

We are conscious that in addressing issues relating to 'race' and ethnicity many nurses feel uncomfortable and unsure. Still others, in the context of ever-increasing pressures on the profession, may resent what they see as the additional burden of 'political correctness' placed on an already overcrowded and demanding professional agenda. We are also conscious, however, that many nurses are in the forefront of the struggle for better services for minority ethnic communities and have a genuine desire to improve and develop the care they provide. In this book, we hope to show that a greater awareness of 'race' and ethnicity is vital in achieving the fundamental clinical and ethical goals of good nursing practice.

PART I

Ethnicity and health

1 Sociological theories of 'race' and ethnicity

Jon Mulholland and Simon Dyson

Introduction

'Race' and ethnicity are terms widely used within academic, professional and popular language. Yet at the same time, both their meaning, and the nature of the 'realities' to which they refer, remain the subject of confusion and controversy. Despite this, a striking feature of 'race' and ethnicity as features of social, professional and personal life, remains their taken for granted nature as a form of 'common-sense'. Sociological approaches to 'race' and ethnicity emphasize the need to challenge such 'common-sense' understandings as a means to enabling a critical awareness of the complex and dynamic roles played by 'race' and ethnicity within social, political and professional life.

The dynamics of 'race' and ethnicity play an important role in shaping health inequalities, illness behaviour, health care experience and the roles of professional practitioners (Smaje 1996). Health care services within Britain, and the professional groups charged with responsibility for delivering those services, have been slow to incorporate an analysis of 'race' and ethnicity into their theory and practice (Gerrish *et al.* 1996). In fact, to the degree to which such questions have been addressed, they have tended to be relegated to the periphery as the concerns of a minority of clients and an interest of professional specialists. The aim of this chapter is to provide an introduction to sociological approaches to the questions of 'race' and ethnicity. In the process, questions of 'race' and ethnicity will be shown to be central to the very nature of health and nursing care.

The chapter examines the origins of 'racial' theory, accounts for the influence of science in the formation of such theory, and explores its scientific and social scientific critique. Contemporary sociological approaches to 'race' are then reviewed and their limitations considered. We will then look at how the concept of ethnicity has recently been taken up again by sociologists but at the same time has been reworked to reflect the changing nature of society. The implications of these complex theoretical transformations for nursing will be addressed throughout the chapter.

'Race' and scientific racism

Although the idea of 'race' dates back to the sixteenth century, it was not until the eighteenth and nineteenth centuries that 'race' became the explicit focus of scientific attention (Miles 1989, 1993). By the late nineteenth century, a whole scientific body of thought had been constructed within European science regarding the supposedly 'racial' nature of human populations, their capacities and their interrelations. This thinking has come to be known as 'scientific racism'.

Although scientific racism refers to an evolving, complex and contradictory body of thought, some key components may be identified.

- Scientific racism was characterized by a commitment to 'biological reductionism', namely the view that complex wholes, in this case social groups and human populations, may be understood through a process of reduction to their most elementary biological forms. As such, human behaviour, intelligence, and the capacity for civilization and culture were seen as a product of some underlying biological essence, made visible principally through features such as skin colour.
- Humanity was comprised of 'racial' types with fixed yet fundamentally unequal anatomical and physiological characteristics. Furthermore these supposed 'types' were organized in a hierarchy. The alleged 'proof' of the existence of these 'racial types' ranked hierarchically was thought to be the unequal distribution of economic and political power. 'Racial' theories were advanced not only to differentiate European 'races' from the non-European 'other', but also to distinguish between European 'races'.

● The notion that human beings are descended from many different origins was advanced to partially account for the existence of 'racial' differences, challenging the idea that we are all, black or white, ultimately descended from the same people (a principle underlying Christianity's world view).

● Hostility was seen to inevitably characterize the nature of inter-'racial' relations, reflecting natural mechanisms for ensuring the purity of the 'racial' blood stock. As such, sexual intercourse between supposedly different 'races' was generally viewed as spelling potential catastrophe for 'racial' and national health, and was little better for the individual.

As with theoretical/scientific knowledge generally, racial theories did not remain exclusive to the academic community. Rather, they gradually moved into popular culture and political ideology. The assumption that there were biologically different 'races' became a part of the academic/scientific and popular 'common-sense' (Rose and Rose 1986).

A critique of scientific racism has become the starting point for sociological analyses of 'race'. Contemporary developments within genetics do not support the existence of 'races'. For instance, genes associated with one particular trait, such as skin colour, are not linked directly to genes associated with other traits, such as height. Furthermore, 85 per cent of genetic variations in the human population exist on the level of the individual (Jones 1991, Rose *et al.* 1984). Because of this, genetic variation *within* a group will be greater than that commonly found *between* groups. It also means that there is less genetic variation in the human species than is typically found in other species. Moreover, there is no convincing evidence to suggest that there is a link between genetic variation and intellectual and socio-cultural capacities. It is this challenge to the material reality of 'race' as a biological fact, that motivates many within sociology to place the term 'race' within inverted commas, indicating a determination not to create a form of reality where it does not exist (Miles 1982). Scientific racism suggests that unequal power relations between different 'races' are inevitable and unchangeable because they are biologically determined. Sociologists suggest that power relations are social issues that do not occur naturally, are not inevitable and can be changed.

Despite the discrediting of 'racial' theory, there are a number of reasons for thinking that biologically grounded ideas of 'race' are far from extinct. First, sociobiology, the agenda of which is to explain all social behaviour in terms of an overarching biological explanation (Rose and Rose 1986), has experienced something of an academic revival in recent years. While sociobiology is not inherently racist, its attempts to explain social behaviour in biological terms leave it open to interpretations that could be used to support the notion of distinct biological 'races'. Second, on the level of popular culture, one may also detect assumptions of biological 'race' in the advertising campaigns of companies such as Benetton (Solomos and Back 1996). Through the incorporation of images of black and white children, Benetton symbolizes unity and happiness. But the unity and happiness is a bridge across permanent and unchanging differences between supposedly separate 'races'. The advertisement therefore reinforces biological notions of 'race' rather than challenging them. Third, the hostility towards 'mixed race' relationships (Frankenberg 1993) suggests that deep down many people still think in terms of fixed biological 'races'. The implication is that you can only be concerned about 'mixing races' if you believe in fixed biological 'races' in the first place. Finally, in politics, numerous far-right political groups throughout Europe subscribe to variants of 'scientific racism'.

The critique of scientific racism is particularly relevant for nurses. The biomedical paradigm, widely acknowledged as influential within areas of nursing theory and practice (Mulholland 1995; Holmes 1990), is underpinned by a form of biological reductionism common to that found within biological notions of 'race'. In this sense, biomedicine makes it possible to slip into thinking in terms of biological notions of 'race'. Given the genetic basis of conditions such as sickle cell anaemia and thalassaemia (Anionwu 1993), and their prevalence within groups historically defined in 'racial' terms, there is the danger that 'race' may seem an 'obvious' explanation for making sense of such disease patterns. Moreover, to the degree that 'racial' theory is (wrongly) thought to be credible as an explanation of specific genetic conditions, there is the danger that such theory may 'leak out' and be used to try to explain any or all differences in health outcomes between ethnic groups. There is perhaps less danger that nurses today will base their practice on crude assumptions of biological 'race'. But there is a continuing danger that 'races' will be used as a shorthand way of referring to the process of nursing supposedly distinctive cultural groups.

'Race' without biology

Although 'race' has no material reality in nature, sociological approaches have tended to start from the premise that 'race' becomes real to the degree to which people believe it to be so, and act on the basis of this assumption. The task therefore has been to understand the emergence and prevalence of racial/racist ideologies, practices and outcomes in relation to the broader socio-political and economic context.

John Rex (1970, 1986) adopts an approach influenced by the work of Max Weber, in which he seeks to understand 'race relations' as a product of particular forms of class competition for scarce resources (housing, employment, etc.). He argues that colonialism provided the source of the 'stigmatization' of black migrants in Britain, and that 'racial' consciousness and racism are the product of a white working class struggling for control of employment and housing against a black underclass perceived as an outside threat. It is the allocation of black people to poor occupational positions and their political exclusion that maintains their underclass status. 'Racial' ideas emerge and prevail within such contexts.

Marxists have not understood 'race' as a taken-for-granted starting point, but rather have seen the (false) idea of 'race' as an outcome of racism, racism being seen as an ideology and/or a means of exploiting or excluding people. With few exceptions (Gabriel and Ben-Tovim 1978), Marxist analyses take as their point of departure the view that questions of 'race' and ethnicity cannot be understood in isolation from the broader context provided by the capitalist relations of production, and so seek to understand 'race' within a 'grand' or overarching theory.

For some Marxists (Cox 1948) racism served a function for the capitalist system as a whole. It served to divide the working class and in so doing fragment its economic and political power. As a result capitalists could exploit the black working class to an even greater extent than the white working class.

More recent Marxist writings (Miles 1982, 1989, 1993), claim that 'race' is an ideological construction, a form of false consciousness, and as such cannot be a real object of analysis. For Miles, 'race' can only be understood as a product of those variables that have been causally significant in its genesis, evolution and function.

It is on this basis that Miles is opposed to a sociology of 'race' relations. This is because referring to 'relations' falsely implies that the category 'race' has a basis in reality. This has political dangers because an apparently positive idea of 'good relations' actually reinforces ideas of biologically based difference. In contrast, Miles suggests a sociology of racism as a study of the process of racialization. Racialization in turn refers to '. . . a process of delineation of group boundaries and an allocation of persons within those boundaries by primary reference to (supposedly) inherent and/or biological (usually phenotypical) characteristics' (Miles 1982: 157). Within a racialized ideology, these boundaries are constructed as fixed and the relationship between ascribed 'racial' groups is understood as hierarchical. Miles suggests that racialization is a process inextricably connected to the emergence of capitalist relations of production, and functions as a means of regulation and management. 'Racial' differentiation and consciousness are a product of societies characterized by class conflict, and serve to fragment the working class. As such, there can be no positive role for the 'race' concept, and its usage must cease.

A central achievement of the Marxist tradition has been its insistence that 'race' and racism may only be understood in the context of broader socio-economic and political dynamics. For nurses, who have had a tendency to formulate questions of 'race' and racism as cases of individual prejudice, such a relocating of the problem may serve to open up new avenues for reflection and intervention, particularly with regard to the structural determinants of service provision. As Gerrish *et al.* (1996) imply, an awareness of the impact of personal racism upon practice is necessary, but by no means sufficient, in ensuring appropriate and equitable provision for all in a multi-ethnic society.

New racism, multiculturalism and anti-racism

During the 1970s and the 1980s three different theoretical perspectives on questions of 'race' and ethnicity can be identified. First, 'new racist' ideologies mainly associated with the political right. Second, 'multicultural' perspectives which sought to give value to the ethnic differences to which new racism referred. Third, 'anti-racism' which sought to locate the 'problem' of ethnic diversity within an analysis of racism and discrimination. We now look at each of these in turn.

New racism

The term New Right is not a united whole but a partial alliance of single issue interest groups campaigning on matters as varied as immigration, censorship and sex education (Durham 1991). These groups find common ground only in relation to specific policy questions, one of which has been the 'multicultural society'. The 'multicultural society' is partly the 'problem' and partly the idea against which the New Right comes to define its own political ideology.

New Right interventions in the field of 'race' and ethnicity have been criticized as a 'new racism' (Barker 1981; Gilroy 1987). New racism is different from old racism in that it does not explicitly refer to differences based on biological race, but on differences in culture. 'Races' become reworded as ethnic groups that have fixed cultural differences that are incompatible with one another.

In part, 'race' became transformed into ethnicity as a response to the changing nature of British society. As Cesarani (1996) has pointed out, the 1971 Immigration Act effectively eliminated 'primary' immigration and as a consequence attention has been diverted from the highly racialized boundary between the white and black 'worlds', towards the cultural claims currently being made by Britain's established ethnic minorities. New racism has served to construct minority ethnic groups as impossible for the majority to incorporate because minority ethnic groups are inherently different, inherently outsiders. However, as Solomos and Back (1996) point out, the words may be of culture and ethnicity, but this is really only a coded way of referring to assumed biologically based differences.

New racism thinks of cultures as evolving slowly according to their own logic and within relatively self-contained boundaries, living alongside other slowly evolving cultures (Scruton 1986). From this approach, a culture contains an essence, an inner-secret known only to those with a long-standing experience of it. In other words, those who truly 'belong', have an intuitive awareness of a shared collective memory from which others (racial/ethnic minorities) are excluded. As with the biological theories discussed earlier, individuals are understood as being located within bounded groups, membership of which is inherited, and is seen to determine and set limits on what an individual can be and do.

New racism views prejudice as both 'natural' and universal, reflecting a deep-seated 'racial' sense of belonging, and an inborn hostility to those who are different in these terms. By treating prejudice as something that automatically happens everywhere, new racism implies that racism is natural and normal. The ideas of the New Right have served to construct and consolidate 'common-sense' notions of culture and ethnicity as coded referents to 'race'. Ideas that minority ethnic patients require 'special treatment' reflects the manner in which the needs of such clients are defined as different or 'other'. This in turn is a product of the way in which the NHS is defined as part of British culture. But since no-one defines what is meant by British culture this allows those delivering the service great flexibility. A nurse can regard some variation as within the realms of 'normal' practice (visitors allowed to bring their white patient grapes) and other variations as a request for special treatment (visitors resented for bringing onto the ward food for an ethnic minority patient). Thus ethnic minority clients are judged against conventions that are rarely made explicit. Ethnic minority nursing staff, including Irish, suffer widespread discrimination (Pudney and Shields 1997; Wedderburn Tate 1996; Mensah 1996), even though, as we shall see in Chapter 11 by

Culley *et al.* on Caribbean nurses, they have made substantial contributions to the NHS. Taken together, these two factors (discrimination against ethnic minority patients and discrimination against ethnic minority staff) may in part be understood in terms of a new racism that constructs the NHS as a racialized British cultural 'space'.

Multiculturalism and the 'classical' model of ethnicity

In the 1970s and the 1980s multiculturalism sought less to challenge the idea of ethnic-cultural difference constructed by the New Right, and more to reverse the evaluations of such differences, to replace the negatives with positives. Its central aim was to construct a pluralistic society within which distinct ethnic communities may reside in mutual harmony, understanding and acceptance. The worrying similarities between new racist and multicultural conceptions of ethnic difference reflects their common adherence to a 'classical' model of ethnicity.

In referring to a 'classical' model of ethnicity underpinning the multiculturalist projects of the 1970s and the 1980s, it is important to emphasize that understandings of ethnicity tended to be implicit and taken for granted. However, the following definition of an 'ethnos', or ethnic group, encapsulates the model of ethnicity found within multiculturalism: '. . . a historically formed community of people characterised by common, relatively stable cultural features, certain distinctive psychological traits, and the consciousness of their unity as distinguished from other similar communities' (Bromley 1974: 66). To this initial definition were added the criteria of common territory and a name identifying the group (Bromley 1974). The emphasis is upon the understanding of a stable and resilient set of *core* cultural characteristics.

Anti-racism and the critique of multiculturalism – implications for models of ethnicity

The multicultural approach has been subject to extensive critique, both in its theoretical assumptions and political implications. Anti-racism comes into existence as a critique of multiculturalism. We will now review some of the key elements of this critique.

First, Miles (1982) challenges the widespread way in which culture and ethnicity, which are actually two distinct things, are treated as if they were one and the same thing. Commenting on the work of Wallman (1979), he points out that ethnicity models rarely identify criteria through which to pick out those aspects of culture that are to count specifically as ethnic. For instance, it may be possible to talk of the culture of nursing or medical culture (and indeed to identify and challenge the racism that partly underpins such cultures), but it makes no sense to speak of the ethnicity of nursing or medicine.

Second, ethnicity has wrongly been used in a way that treats culture as if it had a solid existence independent from the socio-political context that helps to create the culture. Ahmad (1993) and Miles (1982: 67) argue that ethnicity has been misused as a key factor shaping human behaviours by inappropriately considering it as an abstraction, independent from broader socio-political and economic relations. Instead we need to give an account of the impact of material deprivation in structuring the way in which ethnicity is experienced.

Such a criticism has been made of the 'transcultural theory' tradition within nursing. Here, ethnic groups have tended to be constructed as essentially cultural communities. Ethnic groups have wrongly been thought of as (1) being made up of people who are all the same, (2) never changing their characteristics, and (3) as having differences that are more important than their similarities to other ethnic groups (Mulholland 1995). The aim of transcultural nursing has been to develop a technical cultural knowledge enabling the transcendence of the cultural divide between nurse and patient (Leininger 1991). However, the effect has been to generate an approach to nursing within a multiethnic society characterized by the construction of static ethnic typologies. Culley (1997) has pointed out that such 'cultural essentialism' is a broader feature of nurse education as a whole. In constructing such an essentialist model, the way in which ethnicity is socially constructed, and can be moulded and interpreted by individual actions, is lost.

The 'ethnic studies' approach has failed to address the manner in which ethnicity is cut across by other dimensions of inequality, such as gender, class, age, and sexuality (Anthias 1998). This has commonly led to treating ethnic groups, which are made up of a wide variety of people, as if the individual people making up the group were somehow all alike. The ethnic studies approach has also led to treating ethnicity as the key causal determinant of human behaviour, thereby disregarding the role played by social class, gender, sexuality, etc. The *Stop Rickets Campaign* and the *Asian Mother and Baby Campaign* of the 1980s have commonly been presented as cases in point. Gerrish *et al.* (1996) have also pointed to the need for nursing to work with a model of ethnicity that recognizes that ethnic groups are made up of people who have differences of class, gender, sexual orientation and age.

One consequence of emphasizing ethnicity has been a certain victimization of minority ethnic groups with respect to the disadvantages they experience (Stubbs 1993; Sheldon and Parker 1992). If ethnicity refers to an individual/group's cultural practices, and if ethnicity is overwhelmingly significant as a causal influence on human behaviour, then it follows that these practices must account for the inequalities in life chances and health outcomes. As a consequence this closes down the possibility of understanding the role played by external forces in shaping life chances and experiences. Bowler (1993a) demonstrated the prevalence of cultural essentialism, and practices of stereotyping and victimization, within her study of midwifery practice and 'South Asian' clients. Pathologizing stereotypes of South Asian clients held by the midwives served to determine the moral value of clients and the quality of care they received.

According to Smaje (1996), ethnicity, when referred to in health research, is commonly treated as a 'left over' category. In other words ethnicity is the explanation given of health patterns as the only thing left when other possible causes such as class, income, employment, marriage patterns have been ruled out. This is unsatisfactory in two ways. First, this defines ethnicity in terms of what it is not, rather than what it is. And second, this still does not tell us anything about the mechanisms by which ethnicity may be causing the patterns of health under investigation.

The notion of an ethnic group characterized by a common commitment to a shared and stable cultural 'core', as expressed in the work of Bromley (1989), and underpinning 'common-sense' notions of ethnicity, has been extensively challenged

(Jenkins 1997). Even if we acknowledged the existence of ethnic groups, and the existence of shared cultural practices, what is to prevent their interaction with the broader socio-economic climate bringing about fundamental changes to cultural practices and identities to the point that the very existence of a stable core is questioned?

Much research into ethnicity has been criticized for its focus upon the 'exotic'. By this is meant a focus upon those attributes (often more the product of racist ascription on the part of the observer) that are seen as defining 'their' difference or 'otherness' (Stubbs 1993). The preoccupation with issues of diet and dress within stereotypes of minority ethnic groups would serve as an example. It is this notion of ethnicity, and its association with 'exotic' difference, that explains why majority populations often do not think about their own ethnicity. From such a vantage point, they do not appear to have one. Frankenberg (1993) usefully points out that we need to explore what 'whiteness' actually means. If the cultural practices that the term 'white' refers to remain unnamed it means they cannot be challenged. If they cannot be challenged then 'whiteness' as a racialized identity gives that group a structural power advantage.

Central to the anti-racist critique of the 'ethnicity paradigm' was its general failure to address the questions of power, 'race' and racism (Jenkins 1997; Banks 1996). Anti-racism claimed to understand those social phenomena (and their dynamics) commonly labelled as ethnic, not in terms of culture, but by reference to concepts such as ideology and power, 'race' and racism. The creation of the 'good' society required, from an anti-racist standpoint, a political and social unity in struggle against oppression. This helps explain the emergence of the idea of the 'political colour of blackness' in the late 1970s and the 1980s. This involved using the term 'black', not as a description of the colour of a person's skin, but rather as a political category marking a population unified by its common experience of racism.

New directions

The anti-racist position, while offering an invaluable critique of both new racism and multiculturalism approaches has itself been challenged in recent years. These criticisms have included:

- Anti-racism treats the concept 'race' as a taken-for-granted starting point rather than explaining how its widespread use as a term has come about in social, political and historical terms.
- Anti-racism also ends up treating groups as fixed, unchanging with no blurring of boundaries.
- Anti-racism does not go beyond a critique of racism and provide a positive model of the 'multiracial' society.
- Modood (1990) has suggested that the political concept of blackness ignores important ethnic differences between Asian and African-Caribbean populations.
- Modood (1990) also argues that anti-racism attaches too much significance to the experiences of racism in determining identities, interests and what groups people feel they belong to on socio-political issues.

Black feminism

From the vantage point of black women's experiences, black feminism has challenged sociological theories of 'race', particularly those underpinning anti-racism. Fundamental to this challenge has been the claim that sociological conceptualizations of 'race' have failed to account for the multiple and interactive nature of oppression (Anthias 1998; Frankenberg 1993; Hill-Collins 1991; bell hooks 1989; King 1988). Black women's lives illustrate that we are all located at the intersection of diverse 'dimensions of oppression' ('race', class, gender, age). How these different sets of social relations interact is difficult to predict, and can only be understood in relation to specific historical contexts (Frankenberg 1993). The struggle against one mode of oppression in no way guarantees the alleviation of oppression generally.

The socio-political identity and interests of people is not dictated by any one single discourse or set of material relations. The human subject is fragmented and complex, reflecting the nature of the social world, and the relevance of 'race' to a person's life varies over time and is dependent upon the particular context. For instance, a black male nurse may potentially experience a relative disempowerment in relation to a white female patient on the basis of their 'race', yet experience relative empowerment on the basis of their gender and 'expertise'. There is no 'primary' or principal mode of oppression, and as such we need to discard binary models of power which assume that in all contexts there are only two constituencies, the powerful and the powerless (white/black, men/women, young/old, expert/lay). The black feminist emphasis upon the complex and multidimensional nature of oppression also serves to challenge the 'essentializing' of black/minority ethnic clients in terms of their 'racial'/ethnic identity.

The return to ethnicity

Several factors (both analytical and empirical) have led to a 're-discovery of ethnicity' within sociology (Solomos and Back 1996). These factors include (1) the centrality of culture and ethnicity to contemporary racism, (2) the role played by claims to ethnicity as a basis for political mobilization and solidarity, (3) the emergence of 'new ethnicities' within a social context marked by diversity and change, and (4) the influence of postmodernist emphases on questions of culture and identity.

Several authors have argued for a reinstatement of ethnicity within sociological analyses (Modood 1990; Smaje 1997; Hall 1996a, 1996b; Gilroy 1993, 1997; Anthias and Yuval Davis 1992). To varying degrees, such work reflects the influence of Frederick Barth (1969).

Barth (1969) argued that ethnicity is a social construction. Ethnicity, or more specifically, the particular forms taken by an ethnic group, have no predetermined or 'given' nature. According to Cohen (1974), this marks a shift away from understanding ethnicity in terms of its social structure or organizational forms (as if it was an object to be studied) and towards an understanding ethnicity as a *process* (as if it was something that people actively created through practice). Barth is therefore opposed to any approach to understanding and describing ethnicity that focuses upon the supposed content of an ethnic group in terms of some typology of linguistic, religious, cultural and 'diet and dress' characteristics.

Ethnicity is about the relationship *between* groups. Ethnic identities only exist in their relationships to others. Marking ethnic boundaries is a dynamic process and is a product of the ways in which groups construct difference through both self-identification and categorization by others.

Ethnicity, diaspora and hybridity

The term diaspora has become central to many contemporary approaches to understanding ethnicity. By diaspora, we mean 'a network of people, scattered in a process of non-voluntary displacement, usually created by violence or under threat of violence or death. Diaspora consciousness highlights the tensions between common bonds created by shared origins and other ties arising from the process of dispersal and the obligation to remember a life prior to flight or kidnap' (Gilroy 1997: 328). Therefore, on one level, diaspora refers to processes of mass migration, to the global dispersion of populations (Cohen 1979) such as that evidenced by the postwar migration of people from Africa, the Caribbean and the Indian subcontinent to the British Isles. However, on another level, diaspora describes a social condition and a particular type of 'consciousness' (Gilroy 1997) created in the process of migration and movement. Diaspora and diaspora consciousness, rather than being the isolated and exceptional experience of the few, increasingly come to define the times through which we are living. They demonstrate the need to move beyond a 'common-sense' notion of ethnic groups. Ethnic groups can no longer simply be thought of as social groupings living within specific territories, who have existed there from the beginning of human history, and who possess a core set of cultural characteristics that do not change over time.

Gilroy (1997) claims that diaspora illustrates that ethnic identity is continually constructed and reconstructed within changing historical contexts, albeit using the raw materials of what went before (tradition). Gilroy suggests that there is a constant interplay between the past and the present but in such a way that the past is itself rewritten in its application to the present. Gilroy uses the concept *the changing same* to describe this process. For instance, in the context of nursing practice, such a model would suggest the need to understand the ethnicity and health care needs of a young British women with a South Asian family background as being significantly different to those of her mother and grandmother. In contrast to the way in which those of South Asian descent are treated within health care arenas as if they all have the same needs and experiences, the concept of diaspora highlights the dynamic roles taken by 'tradition', migration experience and national and local contexts in the formation of diverse ethnic identifications.

It is not merely that ethnicities change over time that is significant, but also that their respective developments can no longer be understood as being separate or self-contained. According to Barker (1998), the presence of Asian populations in Britain has fundamentally altered the development of both Asian and non-Asian British groups. The contemporary reality of ever increasing diversity highlights the essentially *hybrid* nature of ethnicities. In other words, the various processes of ethnic identification that are going on cross over and mix with one another. Traditions and cultural practices come into close contact with other traditions and practices. Ethnic identities transform in interaction with one another, incorporating, discarding and 'inventing' new cultural practices. As such, hybridity has been presented as undermining ethnic essentialisms. The manner in which some nurses stereotype minority ethnic clients may be a consequence of treating cultures as a fixed series of facts to be learned (the multiculturalist understanding of ethnicity that is currently valued within health service provision). This thinking about cultures in a fixed way then gets in the way of the reality of ethnic complexity and fluidity, and the need for flexibility in thinking during the process of nursing. This also suggests a potential way in which educational initiatives could challenge such stereotyping. This would be to focus upon how different processes of forming identities mix together and cross over with one another.

However, while recent social theory is concerned with the potential for ethnic identities to be thought of as fluid, in certain political contexts ethnic identities are being treated as fixed and absolute. Solomos and Back (1996) point out that the contemporary era is marked as much by the rise of ethnic absolutism, as evidenced in contexts as diverse as Israel, Kosovo and Ireland. This ought to qualify any attempt we might make to equate globalization and crossing over with the end of aggressive and exclusive ethnic absolutisms, or the widespread nature of less violent forms of ethnocentrism and ethnic stereotyping.

Ethnicity, identity and identification

Central to questions of both 'race' and ethnicity is the problem of identity. According to Gilroy (1997: 301), identity offers a way of understanding the '. . . interplay between our subjective experience of the world and the cultural and historical settings in which that fragile subjectivity is formed'. However, when we identify ourselves, or are identified by others, in 'racial' or ethnic terms, what are we to make of such identities? According to Barker (1998), Hall places together two distinct ways of thinking about identity. Underpinning much of Western thought in the last 500 years (including most sociological and anthropological work) has been a model of the human subject as possessing an identity determined by some 'real' essence inherent within that individual, or the social group to which they belong. This essence in turn reflects forces (in nature or in society) that serve to structure the subject's identity. The human subject or self is therefore understood as a 'unified whole', because it is entirely taken over by this essence. For instance, within an 'essentialist' framework, a man's masculinity may be taken to define his very nature, shaping his sense of self, his sexuality, his value-system, his mannerisms and so on. There is no part of him not taken over by his masculinity. Likewise, essentialist models of ethnicity treat individual identities as merely specific examples of a broader ethnic type.

Hall (1990) suggests an alternative way of conceptualizing identity, namely the 'postmodern' approach, which presents a view of contemporary society as having entered a postmodern stage of development. If the modern period (arguably dating from the Enlightenment to the postwar period) was marked by scientific certainty, the formation and consolidation of nation-states, and mass political mobilization around stable social identities, the postmodern period marks its very opposite. The latter is characterized by a general 'crisis' in all of these realms. The ever increasing difference and diversity of social life has fundamentally destabilized society and removed the certainties that previously governed personal and social relations. The consequence is a society marked by a radical and far-reaching diversity of identities in social, economic and cultural life. According to Hall (1996b), a process of globalization has been pivotal in bringing about such destabilization and change.

This 'postmodern condition' of continuous change, ever increasing diversity and moral relativity has prompted questions as to the validity and utility of our existing conceptual and theoretical concepts for understanding social life (Rattansi 1994; Smart 1983). Postmodernist approaches attempt to challenge ideas that identities are made up of fixed essences. Rather postmodern approaches think of the human subject a bit like a hologram. A hologram is nothing more than the temporary effect we get as a by-product of different sources of light shining into a particular space. For postmodern thinkers our identities are seen not as fixed but as the outcome of several sets of competing and contradictory sets of ideas and social relations. The process whereby a given person comes to identify with a particular social identity cannot be taken for granted and certainly not predicted. Nurses cannot therefore assume in advance whether the most important influence on a patient's care will be their nationality, their food preferences, their kinship relations, their religion, their skin colour, their gender, their age, their sexual orientation, their socio-economic background or whatever. Only by carefully asking the patient to express their needs in their own terms can nurses adequately work competently with the different and complex identities of their clients. Such an insight undermines the stable conceptual categories commonly utilized in the analysis of 'culturally sensitive nursing care'. Which processes of identification are temporarily central to a patient's identity will vary over time and between contexts.

As Hall (1996a) points out, even the term identity implies a self that is formed, unified and stable. It is for this reason that

Hall (1996a) suggests 'identification' as a more appropriate way of understanding questions of ethnicity. The important distinction here is the shift from understanding ethnicity not as something that you *are* or *have*, but rather as something that you *do*. Ethnicity represents a *process* of identification; an unstable and ongoing process of constructing an ethnic identity out of the historical resources available. To paraphrase Hall, ethnicity is not so much *what we are* as *what we might be*. One way of thinking about culturally competent nursing is therefore as helping the patient to *become* what they want to be.

According to Hall (1996b), identification is a product of boundary construction, through which we come to mark certain differences as ethnically important and others as not. Identification has important broader consequences for the way we live our lives because our ethnic identity becomes constructed in the process of excluding that which we are not. Those symbols, or 'border guards' (Armstrong 1982), that come to mark the boundaries of social groups are by no means predetermined or given (Anthias and Yuval Davis 1992). They are the product of humans deciding what aspects of life are important in defining who they are. The sense of 'naturalness' that may accompany our ethnic identifications, and the 'sameness' we may feel with others who so identify may appear 'obvious'. But this ignores the way in which such processes of identifying are socially constructed in the context of particular social, economic, political and historical circumstances. This represents perhaps the greatest challenge to a nursing practice charged with a responsibility to ensure the appropriateness and sensitivity of their care to the real, rather than ascribed, needs of their clients.

Conclusion

Sociological theories point to the need for a fundamental reconsideration of popular and 'common-sense' understandings of 'race' and ethnicity. For nursing, this implies a need for far-reaching and critical reflection upon the conceptual underpinnings of nursing theory and practice. The restructuring of the NHS, and the responsibilities placed upon commissioning bodies in meeting the needs of a diverse population, appears to offer potential for more flexible and sensitive approaches to care (Atkin 1996). The incorporation of criteria relating to the preparation of nurses in meeting the needs of minority ethnic clients (UKCC 1989), within the statutory framework of nurse education, also appears to offer such potential (Le Var 1998). However, a systematic implementation of effective responses to the challenges presented to care by ethnic diversity is yet to be realized (Gerrish *et al.* 1996). The potential of any such response is also entirely dependent upon the nature of its theoretical underpinnings.

The need to challenge common-sense notions of 'race' and ethnicity will be central to enabling a more critical evaluation of the impact of such dynamics upon nursing theory and practice. A full appreciation of the discredited nature of biological theories of 'race', and a recognition of the role played by 'race' as a source of group-based identification and ascription would enable nurses to evaluate the role played by ideas of 'race' in the delivery and experience of nursing care, and better address the dynamics of racism. This process requires the location of questions of 'race' and racism within a broader social and political analysis. Ethnicity has become the central concept in thinking about cultural diversity within nursing theory and practice. However, common-sense typologies of ethnic groups, understood as bounded social groupings living within specific territories and characterized by an attachment to a core set of cultural characteristics that goes back to the dawn of time and does not change greatly in the course of history, have tended to predominate within the literature. The usefulness and appropriateness of such typologies is criticized by contemporary sociological approaches to ethnicity. These new approaches emphasize the interactive, complex and fluid nature of ethnic identifications. Such approaches offer a challenge to new forms of cultural racism that take as their starting point the idea of fixed, bounded ethnic groupings that are fundamentally incompatible with one another. They also offer the potential for appreciating an ethnic dimension to patient need and nursing care, but in a manner that incorporates an understanding of the ethnicity of the patient as an identity constantly on the move. It is precisely because of this capacity for ethnic identifications of being transformed and worked on, that effective nursing practice must take as its starting point the positive ethnic identifications of the client, rather than the ascribed characteristics given to them within an ethnocentric 'common-sense'. Of central importance is a greater awareness of the nature in which ethnicity interacts with other dimensions of inequality such as gender, sexuality or class. Finally, only with a recognition that ethnicity comes to be defined at the boundary between 'us' and 'them', will nurses be equipped to explore their own identifications and the manner in which these impact upon their practice.

2 The health status of minority ethnic groups

Simon Dyson and Chris Smaje

Introduction

Chapter 1 considered how boundaries between ethnic groups are not fixed but fluid, changing on the basis of the actions of individuals and the changing material circumstances in which they live their lives. However, ethnic identities are relatively enduring, involving as they do notions of shared ancestry and shared geographical origin, real or imagined (Bradby 1995). These ethnic identities also correlate with particular health experiences (which is not to say that the health experiences are caused by the ethnic identity). In particular a major source of concern for nurses should be the manner in which the health statuses of minority ethnic groups in the UK appear, generally speaking, to be worse than the health status of the white populations (Nazroo 1997a). These inequalities form the focus of the current chapter.

We begin with a consideration of the methodological problems of trying to describe differences in health status between different ethnic groups, noting the limitations of data that rely on premature deaths or self-reported illness as measures of health, and that rely on country of birth as an indicator of ethnicity. We then describe patterns of mortality, examining first overall patterns and then considering deaths from particular causes such as heart disease, strokes and cancers. We next consider evidence concerning self-reported levels of illness, noting how this evidence challenges some assumptions which have guided recent health care interventions, such as the assumed link between coronary heart disease and people of South Asian descent. We then begin to assess critically the major competing theories as to *why* these patterns may exist by looking at the roles of genetics, migration, racism, access to health services, socio-economic and cultural factors in determining health status.

Finally, we look at the issues of social cohesion, social status and social standing as factors that may provide the link between culture and material factors.

Methodological problems

Methodological problems may be compounded by political reasons for lack of data. For example, the health status of those of Irish descent remains especially unknown (Greenslade *et al.* 1997). Those of Irish descent are now overwhelmingly British-born to parents who themselves are British-born (Greenslade *et al.* 1997). As no category for Irish ethnicity was available for use in the 1991 Census, data are restricted largely to figures for mortality based on country of birth (Adelstein *et al.* 1986).

With early data on the health of Asian, African and Caribbean immigrants (Marmot *et al.* 1984) the use of mortality as a measure of health has a number of problems. First, mortality rates for these minority ethnic groups, by virtue of focusing on death, tend to concentrate on older generations and thereby primarily on immigrants rather than British-born ethnic minorities. Second, use of mortality rates tends to understate inequalities. This is because the occupation listed on the death certificate of migrants may be the highest occupational level achieved (perhaps teacher in country of origin) rather than the occupation in Britain (perhaps unskilled factory worker) (Nazroo 1997a) owing to downwards occupational mobility at the time of migration (Nazroo 1998). Third, the country of birth is sometimes not fully identified and even cruder categories such as continent (Africa or Asia) are referred to (Nazroo 1997a). In the case of Irish peoples, using Ireland as country of birth aggregates both Protestant and Catholic from both Northern Ireland and Eire (Greenslade *et al.* 1997).

Other measures present different types of problems. Measures of outpatient attendance or hospitalization rates may depend on problems of access to services and/or differences in rates of presentation of symptoms rather than levels of ill-health. Survey questions depend upon the particular phrasing of the questions asked and the method of sampling used to identify respondents.

Survey questions also rely upon the respondent understanding symptoms, seeking health services, remembering symptoms and/or health service utilization and being prepared to disclose any of this to an interviewer. All these factors may lead to variations between all respondents irrespective of ethnicity. But if different ethnic groups do indeed report health differently in any systematic way then this causes problems for analysis (Nazroo 1997a).

Bearing in mind the different limitations of mortality and morbidity data we now propose to summarize what is known about both death rates and reported illness rates of minority ethnic groups.

Patterns of mortality in minority ethnic groups

Allowing for the methodological problems of data based on country of birth and death rates, we can nevertheless identify certain patterns in rates for both men and women from Ireland, the Indian subcontinent, Africa and the Caribbean.

There are several points worth making about Table 2.1:

- The SMR is the standardized mortality ratio. This measure compares the mortality rates of two populations, taking account of differences in their age structure. The SMRs in the table express age-adjusted death rates for each migrant group as a ratio to the death rates for the whole resident population of England and Wales, which is set by definition at 100. SMRs greater than 100 indicate a higher age-adjusted mortality than this population. SMRs less than 100 indicate a lower age-adjusted mortality than this population.
- Note that the reference group therefore includes all minority ethnic groups resident in England and Wales both those born abroad and those born in England and Wales.
- Remember that the table looks at deaths (and may therefore hide inequalities in levels of illness between ethnic groups) and country of birth (and that this is not the same as ethnic group, as at the 1991 Census about half of the minority ethnic groups in the UK were British born).

Table 2.1 Mortality from all causes by selected place of birth, England and Wales, 20–64 years, adjusted for age and marital status, 1991–93.

		SMR adjusted for age	SMR adjusted for age and marital status
Caribbean	Women	104	94
	Men	89*	78*
African (West/South Africa)	Women	142*	121*
	Men	126*	118*
Indian subcontinent	Women	99	101
	Men	107*	119*
East African (mainly Asian)	Women	127*	126*
	Men	123*	135*
All Ireland	Women	115*	112*
	Men	135*	123*
Scotland	Women	127*	125*
	Men	129*	125*
England and Wales**	Women	100	100
	Men	100	100

* SMR statistically significantly different from 100.
** All people resident in England and Wales.
Source: Adapted from Maxwell and Harding (1998: 21).

- Overall the pattern is one of considerably worse death rates for those born outside England and Wales.
- Note, however, that not all differences are statistically significant.
- Bearing in mind the use of the category 'White' in the 1991 Census, note the especially high relative mortality rates for those born in Ireland and Scotland.
- Note, though, how the degree and in some cases the direction of inequality varies according to gender as well as country of birth. Although not shown here, the inequality also varies according to which age groups within each ethnic group are considered.
- However, in order to prevent misinterpretation of the results, note that SMR values are gender-specific. This means that in theory Caribbean men *could* have higher mortality than Caribbean women despite the lower SMR

value in the table, because the SMR measures mortality against the gender-specific value of the general population (which might be – and in fact is – higher for men than for women).

- Be aware that the Indian subcontinent covers those of Indian, Pakistani and Bangladeshi birth and that other evidence suggests that there are considerable differences between these groups.

- The Caribbean category will include not only those of African descent but also a small number of Indian and Chinese descent whose ancestors came as labourers to the Caribbean in the nineteenth century.

- Marital status is associated with health status (those married typically having improved health status) and is controlled for in the final column. This is important given the very high rates of marriage among those of South Asian descent. However, note that in most instances the majority of the difference between groups remains.

So far the mortality figures we have looked at do not distinguish between different causes of death. Table 2.2 shows that we need to be aware of important differences as well as similarities between death rates for heart disease, cerebrovascular disease and lung cancer.

The figures from Table 2.2 show a very complex pattern but the following points are of note:

- Those born in the Caribbean appear to have higher death rates from cerebrovascular disease, lower rates from lung cancer. Only the Caribbean men, though, have significantly lower death rates from heart disease. Both men and women appear to have lower death rates from lung cancer.

- Those born on the Indian subcontinent appear to have raised risks of death from heart disease and cerebrovascular disease. They appear to have lower death rates from lung cancers.

- Those born in Ireland both men and women have considerably higher death rates from heart disease, cerebrovascular disease and especially lung cancer.

Table 2.2 Standardized mortality ratio (SMR) adjusted for marital status for selected causes, by country or region of birth and sex, 20–64 years, 1991–93.

		SMR adjusted for age and marital status		
		Ischaemic heart disease	Cerebrovascular disease	Lung cancer
Caribbean	Women	92	161*	32*
	Men	54*	145*	53*
Indian subcontinent	Women	173*	135*	34*
	Men	161*	183*	51*
All Ireland	Women	126*	116*	140*
	Men	112*	120*	148*
Scotland	Women	125*	128*	160*
	Men	114*	106	141*
England and Wales**	Women	100	100	100
	Men	100	100	100

* SMR statistically significantly different from 100.
** All people resident in England and Wales.
Source: Adapted from Maxwell and Harding (1998: 21).

- Those born in Scotland, both men and women, have considerably higher death rates from heart disease and especially lung cancer. The raised mortality for cerebrovascular disease is significantly raised for women and raised, although not significantly, for men.
- It is also important to look at absolute rates of mortality as well as relative rates. A small difference in relative rates for a disease that affects many people translates into many more cases than a large difference in relative rates for a disease which affects relatively fewer people. So, for example, ischaemic heart disease probably contributes more to the burden of ill-health for Caribbean men than sickle cell anaemia, even though the relative rates for the latter are much higher than the former. It is these absolute rates rather than the relative ones measured by SMRs, which are of greater importance in planning service provision (Bhopal undated; Bhopal 1988).

Table 2.3 Standardized mortality ratio (SMR) unadjusted for marital status, for selected causes, by country of birth, 20–69 years, 1988–92.

	Diabetes	Hypertensive disease
Other African	230*	697*
Caribbean	436*	460*
India	323*	167*
Pakistan	396*	141
Bangladesh	543*	67
East Africa	221*	147
England and Wales**	100	100

* SMR statistically significantly different from 100.
** All people born in England and Wales.
Source: Adapted from Raleigh *et al.* (1997: 124).

- It is important not to read these figures off from the table as evidence of an 'ethnic' effect as the figures are not controlled for socio-economic status. However, 'ethnicity' never determines health status in and of itself. But the identification of an apparent 'ethnic effect' after controlling for other relevant factors, can help us to bring our hypotheses about possible causal mechanisms into sharper focus.
- The figures for Scotland raise an interesting point. Would we say that there is something genetically different about the Scottish 'race' that leads to premature death? Almost certainly not. We would look to measures of material deprivation and health behaviours. Yet that is precisely this misplaced 'racializing' of health variations in Caribbean and South Asian groups that continues to be a danger in interpreting the figures.

So far the mortality figures we have looked at do not distinguish between different countries on the Indian subcontinent. Table 2.3 shows that we need to be conscious of the differences as well as similarities between death rates for people born in India, Pakistan, Bangladesh or East Africa.

There are several factors to be aware of in interpreting the figures from Table 2.3:

- In this table the figures are for men and women taken together. The table therefore hides potential differences in death rates between sexes as well as between different age cohorts.
- The reference group is those born in England and Wales. Again this will include those of minority ethnic descent born in England and Wales.
- Note, however, the strikingly raised death rates for diabetes for all countries of birth compared to England and Wales.
- Note the extremely high levels of death rates for hypertensive disease relative to the general population for those born in Africa and the Caribbean.
- The figures for India are significantly higher, for East Africa and Pakistan higher, and for Bangladesh lower.

The following table provides figures for a range of causes of death that are, for the first time in this chapter, adjusted for social class. Nazroo (1997a) has argued for the use of direct measures of material deprivation rather than the crude category of class. However, occupational class rather than any direct measure, is what is recorded on the death certificate.

In addition to confirming certain patterns from previous tables we might also note:

- Table 2.4 is controlled for social class but not for marital status. The table also only cites figures for men. It does not look at men of retirement age nor at differences between age cohorts. Death rates may be said to be raised or lowered compared to the general population of England and Wales, which is the reference group here.
- Death rates for heart disease are raised for all migrant groups except Caribbean and West/South African.
- Death rates for cerebrovascular disease are raised for all migrant groups especially Caribbean and West/South African.
- Death rates for lung cancer are raised for Irish and Scottish migrants but are lower for Caribbean and Indian subcontinent migrants.

Table 2.4 Standardized mortality ratios, adjusted for social class, by country of birth, men aged 20–64, England and Wales 1991–93.

	All causes	Ischaemic heart disease	Cerebrovascular disease	Lung cancer	Respiratory disease	Accident and injuries	Suicides
Caribbean	82*	55*	146*	49*	70	109	57
African (West/South Africa)	135*	79	372*	–	–	–	–
East African (mainly Asian)	137*	188*	128	–	162*	104	75
Indian subcontinent	117*	165*	175*	52*	98	87	76*
All Ireland	129*	115*	124*	145*	143*	169*	134*
Scotland	132*	212*	112	151*	142*	184*	160*
All countries**	100	100	100	100	100	100	100

* SMR is statistically significant.
** All men 20–64 resident in England and Wales irrespective of the country in which they were born.
Source: Adapted from Harding and Maxwell (1997: 114, 116, 118, 119).

- Death rates for respiratory disease are raised for Irish and Scottish migrants but are not for Indian subcontinent migrants and may be lower for Caribbean.
- Death rates for accidents are raised for Irish and Scottish migrants but are not significantly different from the reference group for Caribbean and Indian subcontinent migrants.
- Death rates for suicides are raised for Irish and Scottish migrants are lower (though not significantly) for Caribbeans and are significantly lower for Indian subcontinent migrants.

So far in this chapter we have looked at death rates by country of birth. We now look at the other major source of evidence for health variations and that is patterns of morbidity (illness) reported by people from different ethnic groups.

Patterns of morbidity in minority ethnic groups

The latest evidence of morbidity comes from a very large health survey (Nazroo 1997a) in which people were asked to report on their own health. Although relying on reported health, this does have the advantage of being based on ethnic classification directly rather than country of birth or mother's country of birth. It does include information of those of Chinese descent, although the numbers are frequently too small to draw statistically significant conclusions, but it has the disadvantage not only of excluding Irish as an ethnic category, but thereby incorporating a potentially very disadvantaged group into the white category which is then used as the reference point against which other ethnic minority health is assessed.

As with mortality rates the evidence is complex but the following general points may be made:

- The overall inequality in self-reported health for 'ethnic minorities' as a whole hides considerable variation within each ethnic group. Those of Caribbean and especially those of Pakistani/Bangladeshi descent have higher levels of self-reported ill health, and those of Indian and Chinese have

Table 2.5 Percentage of respondents reporting the condition by self-defined ethnic group.

	Self-reported fair/poor health %	Reported heart disease %	Reported hypertension women %	Reported hypertension men %	Reported diabetes %	Reported respiratory symptoms %
White (including Irish)	27	4.2	12	11	1.7	27
Ethnic minorities	32	4.0	12	10	5.7	18
Caribbean	34	3.7	21	13	5.3	23
All South Asian	32	4.2	8	9	6.2	16
Indian/African Asian	27	3.3	6	10	4.7	15
Pakistani Bangladeshi	39	6.0	13	8	8.9	18
Chinese	26	3.0	6	4	3.0	12

Source: Nazroo (1997a: 192–5).

levels at or below the reference white group. On the one hand, the raised level for those of overall 'South Asian' descent hides the very high levels of reported morbidity for Pakistanis/Bangladeshis. On the other hand, it also hides the similar levels of reported ill health between whites and Indians.

● South Asians are frequently alleged to have worse heart health than whites, but this appears to be made up of very high rates among those of Pakistani/Bangladeshi descent (especially the younger age groups) while levels of heart health in Indians appear to be equal to whites. Caribbeans report similar levels of heart health as whites and Chinese better heart health than whites.

● Indian and Chinese ethnic groups report less hypertension than whites; Pakistanis and Bangladeshis about the same but Caribbeans report more. However, there is also a gender effect here. Overall Caribbean people report high levels of hypertension. The overall figure obscures the very much higher levels reported by Caribbean women and the levels reported by Caribbean men which are at or about reported levels by whites.

● Reported diabetes is raised in all minority ethnic groups considered here, being reported variously as high (Chinese), very high (Indian and Caribbean) and extremely high (Pakistani and Bangladeshi).

● Data were not collected on those defining themselves in ethnic terms as Irish. The Irish appear to have low rates of reporting illness, but then high rates of reporting long standing chronic illness and disability. This may imply a lower level of consultation with symptoms when illnesses are at an early stage (Greenslade *et al.* 1997).

Overall, whether the measurement is mortality or morbidity, the health of minority ethnic groups is generally worse though there are important counter-trends both in terms of ethnic categories (Indians), and disease categories (cancers and respiratory diseases). We now turn to a review of some of the explanations that have been utilized to explain these differences in the health of ethnic groups, namely genetic factors, migration, racism, access to health services, socio-economic status and culture and behaviour.

Explaining ethnic patterns in health status

Genetic factors

Rose *et al.* (1984) suggest that there is no scientific basis for the notion of distinct 'racial' groups. There is potentially more genetic variation between two black people than between either one of those two black people and a white person. This is because only a fraction of inherited characteristics are visible (such as skin colour). It makes little sense to say that there is a systematic biological basis to socially ascribed racial or ethnic collectivities. The division of the human species into 'races' on the basis of the incidence of certain types of gene frequencies (associated with traits such as skin colour or hair type) reflect social decisions not an underlying biological classification.

However, a distinction needs to be drawn between arguing for a biological basis to 'racial groups' (which we reject) and the argument that there can be specific genetic factors that are broadly correlated with (that is, associated with but not caused by) some socially ascribed ethnic identities. There is geographical variation within the human species in genetic constitution. However, it is as a result of historical patterns of human contact that socially defined 'racial' classifications also conform to a rough geographical patterning. There is a (highly imperfect) association between social groups who have been given 'racial' labels and some genetic traits.

However, rejecting notions of distinct biological 'racial groups' does not mean completely rejecting genetic factors as possible explanations of health variations between ethnic groups. At the same time, we need to beware of focusing too much on conditions in which genetic factors play a large contributory part such as sickle cell, at the expense of conditions that affect all ethnic groups such as heart disease, hypertension or diabetes (Smaje 1996). To the extent that conditions such as heart disease have any genetic component, such components may be *associated with but not caused by* racialized identities with which social groups are labelled. And we need to recognize that even with this type of partial association between ethnic group and genetic factors, that genes only have an influence in the context of other genes, the whole body, the physical environment and the social environment (Rose 1997).

Migration

Both those of Irish descent, and minority ethnic groups such as those of Caribbean or South Asian descent, have a long history of migration to Britain dating back hundreds of years (Fryer 1984; Greenslade *et al.* 1997). Nevertheless the postwar period saw an expansion of numbers of migrants, generally declining or even reversing from the 1960s onwards. There are at least four possible mechanisms by which migration may have influenced health (Smaje 1995a).

First, there is the *residual* pathway in which adverse health status from the environment of place of origin is 'carried over' into the new life post-migration. An example would be previous poor diet and its continuing influence on later health prospects.

Second, there is the potential for the *process* of migration to affect health negatively. This may occur by the migration process breaking social support networks; by exposing the migrant to stressful situations (exposure to racism as well as general uncertainty as to how to access goods and services required); or by financial commitments, such as the money to pay for the migratory travel in the first place or the kinship obligation to send monies back to relatives in the country of origin.

The third mechanism linking migration and health is *self-selection* in which the healthier person might be relatively more likely to migrate than the less healthy one.

Finally there is the role of *socio-economic* factors in many types of migration. Miles (1982) and Phizacklea (1984) suggest that labour markets needs of capitalism draw in migrant workers specifically to fill poorly paid positions involving long hours and stressful working conditions, exposing them to inner city residence with substandard housing and relative lack of amenities. This draws our attention to the manner in which migrants may be downwardly socially mobile in the process of migration.

In evaluating these respective possibilities, Nazroo (1997a) compares British-born and migrant people from minority ethnic groups. He suggests that overall the health of migrants is at least as good as British-born ethnic minorities of the same age, and may in some instances be better. Broadly speaking, this means that the evidence is against the first possible explanation. In other words, the carry over of negative environmental effects from the country of origin does not appear to explain differences in health statuses of minority ethnic groups in Britain. The evidence on the significance of the processes of migration is difficult to assess. It is even possible that different causes are operating at the same time in opposite directions and partially cancelling out each other.

The evidence appears generally more supportive of the latter two arguments, namely that there is a healthy worker migration selection effect. The evidence from Nazroo (1997a) is also consistent with the socio-economic explanation that emphasizes the direct migration to conditions of poverty, poor environment and racial harassment. This argument is further strengthened by the work of Williams (1993), who suggests that increased length of time in Britain increases the level of poor health among migrants.

In summary, there appear to be higher levels of ill-health among migrants than among the population as a whole. The evidence does not suggest such levels of ill-health are caused by the processes of migration nor by 'carry over' of previous poor health. It does suggest that relatively healthy migrants migrate to work in poorly paid occupations in deprived environments, compounded by facing racism, such that there is a relative decline in their health over time.

However, the effect of migration is linked in complex ways to other factors such as culture, gender imbalances in the migrant population, and utilization of services. As large scale primary immigration has greatly declined, the direct contribution of migration effects to explaining health in all minority ethnic groups, both migrant and British born, will diminish. Nevertheless, broader material, environmental and cultural effects of migration may not disappear straight away, even in generations born in Britain.

Racism

Racism may be said to affect health adversely in three ways (Smaje 1995a). First, through *racism in health service provision and delivery*. Second, there is the *indirect effect of racism* (past or present) in areas of social life in which life chances are known to be linked to health, especially in material and structural factors. And third, there are *the possible direct effects of racism* on health.

In assessing the impact of racism in health services delivery one must be careful not to attribute all bad practice with minority ethnic clients to racism. McNaught (1987) describes a range of possible effects including inaccuracies in patient reception and handling; consultations with poor or no explanations or stereotyping of the patient; pressure to consent to treatment on the basis of inadequate explanation; perceptions of the minority ethnic client as less intelligent or a 'bad' patient; and in terms of health surveillance and diagnosis the use of parameters or behavioural models which are specific to white peoples. Racism is a plausible explanation in each case, but one would need to make explicit comparisons to the manner in which low-income clients or indeed all clients are poorly treated in order to attribute such bad practice specifically to racism.

Racism may also be theoretically linked to poorer health in indirect ways. For example racism in the framing of immigration laws (Sondhi 1987) and social security laws (Gordon and Newnham 1985) and in the implementation of the social security system (Amin and Oppenheim 1992; Atkin and Ahmad 1996) will add to poverty in minority ethnic communities over and above any other socio-economic factors. It will also cause stress from the perceived inequities of such procedures. To the extent that racism is present in addition to socio-economic disadvantage in areas such as education, housing and employment, then these areas of social provision may conceivably also contribute to health inequalities.

At least three studies have sought to establish the plausibility of a direct relationship between exposure to the stressors of racism, internalized anger and high blood pressure. Armstead *et al.* (1989) found that exposure to racist film excerpts raised blood pressures in black US college students. Benzeval *et al.* (1992) found that racial harassment is associated with reported acute illness and that racial harassment in the context of work discrimination is associated with both reported acute illness and reported long standing illnesses. Krieger (1990) found a relationship between those who reported 'keeping quiet about unfair treatment' and reported hypertension in black women. In theory, experiencing discrimination but not reporting it might explain the finding of Nazroo (1997a) that Bangladeshis are less likely than other minority ethnic groups to report racial harassment while at the same time having the highest level of self-reported ill-health.

In summary, racism is intimately bound up with several other explanations for health patterns, especially socio-economic factors and access to services. It may be better to think of racism as underlying and indirect causes on overall ethnic differences in health experience and a potentially significant immediate cause of certain specific outcomes as in the case of a racially motivated physical assault (Smaje 1995a).

Access to services

Ethnic patterns in the use of health services are important in their own right as an index of the quality of service provision, but may also affect health status. There are various possible explanations for different patterns in utilizing health services. In terms of factors influencing clients seeking services these include the health beliefs and knowledge of the population; their knowledge of and attitudes towards health services and what is termed social structure (patterns of kinship, residence, gender relations and social interaction). In terms of the provision of services there is the overall distribution of health care resources; racism in service delivery and quality of care (Smaje 1995a).

Several of these factors are closely associated with, though not reducible to, other explanations such as socio-economic status and racism. Differences in crude rates of service utilization are to be expected on the basis of different age and sex structures of populations (which most studies successfully adjust for) but also on the basis of socio-economic status and patterns of illness (for which most studies have not managed to adequately adjust) (Smaje 1995a). The impact of utilization of services on health status remains therefore difficult to assess. One recent study (Nazroo 1997a) has suggested that

- all ethnic minority groups, except the Chinese, are just as likely as whites to consult a GP;
- when level of self-assessed health are taken into account all ethnic minority groups, except the Chinese, are more likely than whites to consult a GP;
- hospital in-patient rates are at about the same levels as for whites, suggesting that ethnic minority people may be less likely to be admitted to hospital when they have similar rates of illness;
- of particular concern to nurses is that ethnic minority respondents, except for Caribbeans, were less likely to be using health visitors or district nurses.

Issues in the utilization of services are discussed more generally by Smaje (1995a), Smaje and Le Grand (1997) and by Nazroo (1997c).

Materialist explanations

Socio-economic status refers to a range of economic and environmental circumstances that directly affect the social positioning of different ethnic groups and which underlie the ethnic patterning of health status. There are strong positive associations between socio-economic status and health status in the general population. Minority ethnic groups are, in general, associated with lower socio-economic status, and therefore would be expected to have poorer overall health on those grounds. Studies have suggested that ethnic differences in health persist even after taking account of differences in socio-economic status.

However, there are difficulties in measuring socio-economic status across different ethnic groups (Smaje 1995a). First, patterns of residence may be implicated in apparent 'ethnic' differences in disease prevalence. Second, for the same level of income, minority ethnic groups may have less wealth, and therefore less call upon material resources. Third, self-employed people of South Asian descent who are occupationally classified into higher classes may have lifestyles more akin to lower classes (Coronary Prevention Group 1986). Fourth, routine classification of women by their husband's social class is problematic not only for women's health (Arber 1990) but will introduce severe distortions in the analysis of minority ethnic populations where gender differences in social and occupational status are greater still (Ahmad 1994). Social class is therefore problematic because it has variable validity as an analytical concept across different ethnic groups many of whom may not enjoy the same social standing even if they are recorded as being in the same social class (Smaje 1996).

Marmot *et al.* (1984) suggest that social class is a much poorer indicator of mortality among ethnic minorities than for the majority population. However, neither do broader conceptions of material disadvantage such as socio-economic status seem to resolve the issue. For example, 'controlling for socio-economic status' does not itself greatly diminish the relationship between ethnicity and health (Fenton *et al.* 1995; Smaje 1995b). It seems that what is required are more specific and direct measures of material deprivation in order to assess the interaction of ethnicity and material factors in patterning health.

Nazroo (1997a) suggests that various dimensions of material deprivation (such as occupational income, housing tenure, and car ownership) may be exerting a cumulative effect on health. He further argues that for each ethnic group the percentage reporting poor health is linked to (1) whether the households were renting or buying their property, (2) whether there was a full-time worker in the household or not, and (3) whether the occupation was manual or non-manual.

Studies that treat socio-economic status as a confounding variable which is then 'controlled' to leave an allegedly 'true' ethnic effect on health, ignore the explanatory potential of socio-economic status (Nazroo 1997a). Just as racism is likely to leave minority ethnic groups worse off within each social strata (Smaje 1995a), so Nazroo (1997a) provides survey evidence of ethnic variations *within* given levels of income, rates of unemployment and types of housing tenure. He develops a standard of living index based on accommodation (amount of overcrowding), access to amenities (such as indoor toilet) and to consumer durables (such as a refrigerator). He finds that for reported ill-health this standard of living index reduces differences between ethnic groups very significantly in a manner which traditional controls for socio-economic status (class or housing tenure) do not. Furthermore even the standard of living index is a relatively crude measure of deprivation, the implication being that more sophisticated and/or more direct measures of material inequalities may account for the majority of apparent differences in reported ill health between different ethnic groups.

In summary it seems that material deprivation, when measured relatively directly rather than by weak analytical concepts such as class, account for much variation in the reported health status of different ethnic groups. However, deprivation does not explain differences in infant mortality between Pakistani and Bangladeshi babies as both groups are materially disadvantaged (Andrews and Jewson 1993). And even accepting the general strong association does not necessarily tell us about the precise mechanisms which are at work, nor the cultural pathways which may mediate material conditions and health status (Smaje 1995a, 1996).

Culture

In looking at the role of cultural factors in the patterning of the health of different ethnic groups, it is important to develop a dynamic and sophisticated concept of culture and not reduce culture to a collection of health behaviours (Sweeting and West 1995). Early nursing attempts to understand the role of culture in health have been assessed as ethnocentric because they emphasize 'unusual' practices which are then viewed as deviant from the allegedly healthy 'norms' of the ethnic majority (Donovan 1984). Examples include the attempt to 'resocialize-out-of-inappropriate-cultural-practices' ethnocentrism of the *Asian Mother and Baby* campaign of the 1970s (Rocheron 1991) as well as the *Stop Rickets* campaign, campaigns on the use of surma (Pearson 1986a) and consanguinity (Ahmad 1994; Ahmad *et al.* 2000). Ahmad (1996a) identifies several problems with culturalist models of health promotion of this kind.

First, attempts to persuade nurses to learn 'cultures' (e.g. Leininger 1978) ignore the *diversity* within supposedly homogenous cultures. The Bangladeshi community of Tower Hamlets, a relatively undifferentiated community compared to British Pakistanis or British Indians, operate with a complex and overlapping use of Islamic, medical and folk beliefs in constructing their sense of mental illness (Ahmad 1996a; Eade 1995). And James (1993) has noted that it is mainly once in Britain that a single Caribbean identity is created out of the disparate and diverse islands, identities and *ethnicities* of the Caribbean.

Second, the emphasis on cultural difference ignores the extent of *similarities* between different ethnic groups. Third, cultures are not static, but are continually *changing and evolving*. Cultural identity is historically and socially situated, forged in the context of engagement with other ethnicities, including engagement with 'white' ethnicities which themselves are a crude aggregation (Smaje 1996). Fourth, culture is equally a product of *gender, class and other power relations* as much as ethnicity to which it is too often reduced (Ahmad 1996a). Ahmad *et al.* (1989) suggest for example that supposed preference of Asian women for a female GP was on closer examination a preference for a GP who spoke a relevant language. Finally, culture may be a source of *nurturing and strength* (Ahmad 1996a). Thus, for example, it has been suggested that concentration of some minority ethnic groups in certain residential areas may have positive health effects through community integration and social support which may even offset any health damage from the poor material environment often found in the urban areas where minority ethnic groups predominantly live (Smaje 1995b).

The remainder of the chapter should be read with these more complex considerations of culture in mind, and not simplistic conceptions of culture based on victim-blaming or on a narrow range of health behaviours.

Although materialist factors are strongly associated with differences in health statuses of ethnic groups, cultural explanations (although only if they are based on more sophisticated conceptions of culture), may have an explanatory role (Smaje 1996). There is particular potential in examining psychosocial processes (Smaje 1996). These processes act at the level of the individual and their relationships with families and wider communities. These processes may themselves have longer-term consequences of a material nature. Research has begun to examine ethnic patterns in concepts of illness (Anderson *et al.* 1989); the effects of kinship and social networks upon health (Dressler 1988; Brown *et al.* 1992; Williams *et al.* 1992); the importance of religion (Levin 1994) and the impact of cultural context on types of health-related behaviour (Dressler 1993).

However, the effects of cultural variables will crosscut ethnic and social status (i.e. culture will not directly correspond to nor will be reducible to ethnicity). There is a huge variety in background, customs, migration patterns, life histories, social networks, household arrangements and patterns of residence among ethnic groups. The range of this material from which cultural identities may be constructed means that the concepts ethnicity and culture are far from the same thing. The problem is that as we learn more about culture as an explanation of health status, this will not tell us *everything* about ethnicity and it will tell us about factors *other than* ethnicity.

Mediating material factors and culture: social standing

In nursing minority ethnic clients nurses clearly are involved in dealing with the consequences of material social inequalities, which appear strongly linked to health status. There are a limited number of strategies available to nurses, midwives and health visitors to reduce the worst excesses of material deprivation. But what may also be useful is to have a framework within which to think about the potential identities of all clients, including clients from minority ethnic groups.

Rather than thinking of culture as *determining* health behaviours, we need to see that culture may *generate* and *sustain* a varied range of behaviours and attitudes. We do not yet have sufficiently sophisticated concepts understanding how culture is negotiated, changing and enabling rather than limiting and determining behaviour.

Material inequalities are experienced differently depending on how the client puts the possibilities of culture into effect. In turn culture itself is formed in the context of particular material conditions of living (Smaje 1996).

This returns us to a problem we identified earlier. We know that material factors are strongly associated with health status, but not the *mechanisms* by which this association may be played out. In this respect the work of Wilkinson (1996) is instructive. Wilkinson argues that material factors are mediated in a number of ways in affecting health. Each of these factors has implications for the health of minority ethnic groups.

- *Social cohesion* – It is not just the level of material income of a society which determines the health of its population, but the degree to which that income is relatively more or relatively less equally distributed. Moreover, greater levels of material inequality adversely affect not only the disadvantaged but adversely affect the rest of the population as well. This is because material inequality weakens social cohesion generally and leads to a poorer quality of life and greater levels of psychosocial stress for everyone. Inequalities and disadvantages in material conditions, reflected in the poorer levels of health of some minority ethnic groups, diminish the health status of all of us.
- *Social support* – There is evidence for a range of health protecting effects of social support. By social support we mean the amount of control people have over their work; the pressure of work in terms of flow and pace of work; and the degree of emotional sustenance they receive from work relationships. But the importance of feeling in control goes beyond work situations to problems of job or housing insecurity or degree of family conflict. Social support also involves quantity and quality of social contact between people within the home and/or between the

home and wider community. It may involve having a close confiding relationship with a relative, friend or partner. It entails social involvement in the community and participation in quality social networks. Many of these factors involve the degree of control an individual has over her life, and money may itself confer a greater degree of control, all other things being equal. But control of one's life, quality of social support, links to community and confiding relationships mean we have to *interpret* the effect of material factors in producing inequalities in health status. Adverse material conditions may be experienced differently. A cohesive community may partially offset lack of control at the low paid workplace. Family conflict may both exacerbate poor health and itself be a consequence of relative material deprivation.

● *Social status in a hierarchy* – One aspect of the inequalities in health debate we have so far overlooked is that inequalities in health status exist at all levels of income, not just those at the very lowest levels. Wilkinson (1996) links this to chronic psychological stress related to one's social standing in a hierarchy. It is the lower status individuals who are relatively more likely to suffer repeated, chronic and self-reinforcing bouts of heart-damaging steroid hormones released as part of the fight or flight response to distress. The anger, frustration, disappointment of constantly deferring to someone of higher status damages health. But people are part of many social hierarchies, and people from minority ethnic groups may be part of hierarchies based, among other factors, on occupation, income, ethnicity, gender, religion, family, and community standing. These different hierarchies may reinforce one another or alternatively may counteract one another in ways which we do not yet understand.

In this section we have considered how material factors affecting health are mediated by culture, and that culture is itself forged partly in response to particular material conditions. The concepts of social cohesion, social support and social standing may help us to understand the complex ways in which material factors and culture influence each other.

Conclusion

In summarizing complex evidence on the relation between ethnic groups and health status, we may draw a number of tentative conclusions. Genetics may play a large role in some specific disorders (such as sickle cell) and some role in other issues such as heart disease and strokes. However, there are three important cautions with respects to genetics. First, association of certain genetic factors with socially defined ethnic groups is precisely that – an association and not a strong causal explanation of differences in general health status. Second, where this association is treated as a confirmation of a biological basis to race this prevents an investigation of the actual causal factors. Third, genetic factors can in any case only ever influence health in interaction with the whole of an individual's genome, the organism as a whole and the physical and social environment (Rose 1997).

In evaluating the role of migration in determining health status, the explanations of residual ill-health carried over from country of origin and the stresses of the process were not supported by the evidence. The evidence does, however, appear to support the notion that migrants are a self-selected more healthy group. The decline in migrant health over time once in the UK also strongly supports the socio-economic argument that the global economy pulls in immigrant workers to fill certain positions. These positions are in low paid employment in poor working conditions in inner city environments with poor quality housing and a relative lack of local amenities and services. Each of these material factors is associated with poorer health and thus over time the health of some migrants suffers as a consequence of their concentration in such situations.

We have seen that racism contributes to inequalities in health in a few instances directly (such as racially motivated assaults) but more extensively indirectly, by adversely affecting material circumstances of many minority ethnic groups and by the role that racisms have in reinforcing the inequities of social hierarchies.

It has been suggested that some cultural explanations of inequalities in health ignore diversity within minority ethnic groups, overstate cultural differences at the expense of noting similarities in human experiences, do not acknowledge the ever-changing nature of cultures, do not take account of other relations of gender, age and power in constructing culture, do not recognize the health protecting and health nurturing aspects of culture, and do not consider the role of material circumstances in moulding cultures.

Differences are not reducible to social class though, since people from different ethnic minorities may not have the same social standing even if they are recorded as being in the same social class (Smaje 1996). Moreover, the constrained residential options that face minority ethnic groups may themselves influence both health and occupational status. Nevertheless Nazroo (1997a) provides evidence that direct measures of variations in standard of living of different ethnic groups account for a very significant proportion of reported health differences.

However, accepting the strong association between material inequalities and health inequalities does not necessarily tell us about the manner in which relative material deprivation works to affect health status (Smaje 1995a; 1996). Nor does it tell us about the way in which socio-economic conditions are produced and reproduced in different groups. Nor still does it tell us about any ethnic differences in the manner and extent of impact of social roles and social support on health. The work of Wilkinson (1996) suggests that social cohesion, social support and social status in a hierarchy may be the psychosocial *mechanisms* by which material inequalities are associated with health status (note the root cause is still material, the psychosocial is the mechanism). Wilkinson suggests it would be foolish to concentrate interventions on the psychosocial without reducing the underlying extremes of deprivation.

This final point is especially pertinent to nurses, midwives and health visitors whose potential for health interventions at a psychosocial level (offering social support, helping to establish or consolidate social networks) is clearly much greater than their scope for reducing material inequalities. It is important that nurses understand the social context of their care, and in particular the social causes of health inequalities between different ethnic groups. It is also vital that they recognize that their important psychosocial care addresses the *mechanisms* by which material inequalities are experienced by patients and clients.

Nurses therefore need on the one hand to bear witness to the health consequences of material inequalities (and challenge the racism which indirectly pushes some minority ethnic groups into such circumstances). And on the other hand nurses need to recognize that their care interventions will be experienced by clients differently in different material circumstances, in different social networks and at different points of hierarchies of social standing.

3 Ethnic inequalities in mental health

Karen Iley and James Nazroo

Introduction

In this chapter we begin by considering why the area of mental health and minority ethnic groups is likely to be one that raises considerable controversy. We then outline the key findings that have emerged on ethnic differences in mental health. Next, we critically review the sources of data that have produced these findings, allowing the reader to more carefully judge the validity of the conclusions that have been drawn. Following this we review potential explanations for the sometimes contradictory findings that have been published on ethnic inequalities in mental health. This is followed by a discussion of ethnic minority people's experiences of mental health services and the implications this has for mental health care provision and practice. We examine the relative contributions of the sociological concepts of agency and structure for our wider understanding of ethnic inequalities in mental health and the experiences of ethnic minority people in Britain. We conclude with some brief suggestions regarding the practice of mental health nursing.

Controversies

The difference in rates of mental illness among different ethnic groups in Britain is probably one of the most controversial issues in the health inequalities field. This is because it permits a potential link to be made between mental disorders (which are still stigmatized by the general public) and minority ethnic groups (Sashidharan 1993) who, as we have seen, suffer widespread discrimination in many areas of social life. This controversy is made worse by the complexity of conducting research on ethnic differences in mental illness and the consequent disputed nature of research findings. Much of the controversy has focused on the apparently high rates of schizophrenia and other forms of psychosis among the African-Caribbean population, where the possibilities for making (potentially) false links between mental disorder and ethnicity are most apparent. Evidence suggesting low rates of mental illness among the South Asian population, but high rates of suicide and attempted suicide among young South Asian women, has also caused controversy.

Such research evidence on ethnic differences in mental health has, on the whole, been interpreted in one of two ways. It has either been interpreted as an opportunity for further exploration of risk factors for mental illness, through an exploration of the characteristics of those ethnic minorities with higher rates (Nazroo 1998). Or it has been interpreted as a reflection of racism and racist research agendas. Those who have regarded the data on ethnic differences in mental health more critically have focused on the methodological flaws in existing research. First, they have questioned the uncritical acceptance of the data by the majority of the research and policy community. Second they have pointed out how this flawed data conveniently reinforces existing stereotypes about the lives and experiences of ethnic minority people. Third, this reinforcing of racial stereotypes leads to the failure to identify racism as a key component of ethnic minority people's interactions with both psychiatric services and the research community.

Key findings in the literature

There is now an extensive collection of data on ethnic inequalities in health and rapid rise in publications on ethnic differences in the prevalence and experience of illness (e.g., see the review by Smaje (1995a)). It is therefore somewhat surprising that the literature on ethnicity and mental health has largely focused on just two broad groupings: African-Caribbeans and South Asians, and three outcomes: psychotic illness, depression and suicide. The following summary of key findings is structured by these three outcomes, with ethnic groups other than African-Caribbean and South Asian included where possible.

Psychotic illness

Psychotic illnesses, which include schizophrenia, are relatively infrequent. They are thought to affect around one person in 250 (Meltzer *et al.* 1995), but often result in severe disability. Typically they involve a fundamental disruption of thought processes, where the individual suffers from a combination of distressing delusions and hallucinations.

Most research on ethnic differences in psychotic illnesses has been based on treatment rates, and over the past three decades such studies in Britain have consistently shown elevated rates of schizophrenia among African-Caribbean people compared with the white population. African-Caribbean people are typically reported to be three to five times more likely than whites to be admitted to hospital with a first diagnosis of schizophrenia (Bagley 1971; McGovern and Cope 1987; Harrison *et al.* 1988; Littlewood and Lipsedge 1988; Cochrane and Bal 1989; Van Os *et al.* 1996). These findings have been repeated in studies that have looked at first contact with all forms of treatment, rather than just hospital services (King *et al.* 1994), although the rates in one such study were only twice those of the white population (Bhugra *et al.* 1997). Some of the more recent of these studies have also looked at those of African ethnicity and have reported similarly raised rates of psychotic illness in this group (King *et al.* 1994; Van Os *et al.* 1996). Explorations of the demographic characteristics of black people admitted to hospital with a psychotic illness suggest that these illnesses are particularly common among young men (Cochrane and Bal 1989), and some studies have suggested that the rates are very high among young African-Caribbean people who were born in Britain. For example, Harrison *et al.* (1988) report that the rates of first contact with psychiatric services for psychotic illness among this group are 18 times the general population rate.

Given the consistency of the evidence based on treatment statistics, it is somewhat surprising that the only national community based study of mental illness among ethnic minority groups, the Fourth National Survey of Ethnic Minorities (FNS) (Nazroo 1997b), produced rather different findings. Overall, the Caribbean group in that survey did have a raised prevalence of psychotic illness in comparison with the white British group, but not to the level reported elsewhere. For Caribbean people the annual prevalence was fourteen per thousand, in comparison with the rate of eight per thousand for the white group (that is 75 per cent higher in the Caribbean group). And when differences were considered across gender, age and migrant/non-migrant groups it was found that the prevalence of psychotic illness among: men; young men; and non-migrant men; was no greater than that for equivalent white people. For example, the annual prevalence of psychotic disorder among Caribbean men was estimated as ten per thousand while among white British men it was estimated as eight per thousand. The higher rate was exclusively present for Caribbean women.

Findings on rates of psychotic illness among South Asian people are even more mixed. Studies of hospital based treatment suggest that rates of admission for psychotic illness among South Asian people are similar to those among white people (Cochrane and Bal 1989). A more comprehensive prospective study of first contact for schizophrenia with *all* treatment services in one area of London (whose South Asian population is predominantly of Indian origin) confirmed this (Bhugra *et al.* 1997), but an earlier study using the same methods in another London district suggested that rates of psychotic illness among South Asian people (of Indian and Pakistani origin) were raised to similar levels to those found among Black Caribbean people (King *et al.* 1994). Indeed, King *et al.*'s study suggested that rates of psychotic illness among all ethnic minority groups, as defined by the 1991 Census categories, were similarly raised in comparison with a white group, and that among the white people identified as having a first onset of psychotic illness, the majority were not of British origin (King *et al.* 1994). Elsewhere the authors state that 'Most [patients] were from an ethnic minority background, including those people defined as White according to the 1991 Census' (Cole *et al.* 1995: 771). This, of course, suggests that it is misleading to maintain an exclusive focus on those of African-Caribbean origin when examining ethnic differences in psychotic illness. Studies on rates of treatment in hospital have confirmed a possibly high rate of psychosis among those living in England, but born in Ireland (Cochrane and Bal 1989).

In contrast to the findings for contact with treatment services, the community-based FNS prevalence study suggested that rates of psychotic illness might be lower for South Asian people, particularly Bangladeshi people, than those for white British people (Nazroo 1997b). However, when these findings were examined by migration status, it seemed that the lower rates only applied to those South Asians who had migrated to Britain, with non-migrants having rates that were identical to the white British rates. In support of the conclusions drawn by King *et al.* (1994) and Cole *et al.* (1995), the FNS also reported a high rate of psychosis among white people who were not of British origin (they were predominantly, although not exclusively, of Irish origin), who had a 75 per cent higher rate than the white British group.

Depression

Neurotic disorders, which include depression, are much more common than psychotic disorders. A recent national survey suggested that in the week before interview about one person in sixteen was affected by such a disorder (Meltzer *et al.* 1995). They are usefully separated into two categories, anxiety and depression that, although common, do involve considerably more than a sense of anxiety or sadness. Here we will focus on depression, because of the lack of data on ethnic differences in anxiety.

According to treatment statistics, rates of depression among African-Caribbean people appear to be markedly lower than those for white people (Cochrane and Bal 1989; Lloyd 1993), and rates of depression among South Asian people appear to be a little lower than those for white people (Cochrane and Bal 1989; Gilliam *et al.* 1989). For South Asian people, these findings have been confirmed in community studies (Cochrane and Stopes-Roe 1981), including the FNS, which was able to look at those of Indian, Pakistani and Bangladeshi origins separately (Nazroo 1997b). However, as for rates of psychotic illness among South Asian people, further analysis of the FNS by migration status found that the low rates of depression were only found in the migrant group, non-migrant South Asians had the same rates of depression as equivalent white people.

In comparison with the high rates of treatment for psychotic illness among African-Caribbean people, the low rates of treatment for depression are a puzzle. Most factors that might be implicated in the higher rates of psychotic disorders should also lead to a higher rate of other mental illnesses. In addition, in contrast to the low treatment rates, evidence from the FNS suggests that the prevalence of depression among Caribbean people in the community is, in fact, more than 50 per cent higher than that among whites (Nazroo 1997b). Moreover, that study also suggested that despite this higher prevalence, rates of treatment for depression among Caribbean people were very low.

In contrast to the low rates of hospital admission for depression among those born in the Caribbean and South Asia, Cochrane and Bal (1989) reported that rates of admission for depression among those living in England but born in Ireland were markedly higher than for those born and living in England. The high rate of depression among white people who were not of British origin was confirmed in the community based FNS, which reported that this group had rates that were two-thirds higher than the white British group (Nazroo 1997b).

Suicide

In contradiction to the apparent lower overall relative rates of mental illness among South Asian people, analyses of immigrant mortality statistics show that mortality rates from suicide are higher for young women born in South Asia, and this is particularly the case for very young women (aged 15 to 24), where the rate is two to three times the national average (Raleigh *et al.* 1990; Raleigh and Balarajan 1992; Karmi *et al.* 1994). In contrast to the findings for young South Asian women, these studies also showed that men and older women (aged 35 or more) born in South Asia had lower rates of suicide. Analysis of the most recent data on immigrant mortality has been more detailed, because it could be coupled with the 1991 Census which included a question on ethnicity as well as country of birth (Raleigh 1996). This confirmed the overall pattern just described, but showed that the high rates appear to be restricted to those born in India and East Africa.

In terms of morbidity, rather than mortality, a school based study in Birmingham reported very high rates of suicidal ideation (as detected using the General Health Questionnaire) among both male and female South Asians. The authors concluding that 'Suicidal ideation, attempted suicide and suicide are much more common among young Asian women than young white women'. (Merrill *et al.* 1990: 748). In contrast, the only study to look at suicidal thought among a national community population, the FNS, found that the rates of thinking 'that life was not worth living' were similar across South Asian and white groups, lower among South Asian women than white women, and much lower among young (16 to 24) South Asian women (both Indian and Pakistani or Bangladeshi) than young white women (Nazroo 1997b).

Problems with existing sources of data

Although mental illness is a relatively common condition, it is difficult to measure and the defining characteristics are contested. Both the definition and the measurement of mental illness depend on the presence of clusters of psychological symptoms that indicate a degree of personal distress, or that lead to behaviours that cause such distress to others. The clusters of symptoms associated with particular forms of mental illness are clearly defined by psychiatrists (see, e.g., American Psychiatric Association 1995; World Health Organization 1992), although the elicitation of these symptoms for diagnostic or research purposes can be difficult, particularly in cross-cultural studies.

One of the central problems with work on ethnicity and mental illness arises from the reliance of most work on data based on contact with treatment services. Contact with treatment services, even when access is universal as in the NHS, reflects illness behaviour (i.e. the way that symptoms are perceived, evaluated and acted upon), rather than illness *per se* (Blane *et al.* 1996). This raises several linked problems when interpreting differences in treatment rates across ethnic groups, particularly as illness behaviour is likely to be affected by a number of factors that vary by ethnicity, such as socio-economic position, health beliefs, expectations of the sick role and lay referral systems. And these problems become particularly important for work on rates of psychosis, where contact with services might be against the patient's wishes. So, despite the consistency of research findings showing that African-Caribbean people have higher rates of treatment for psychosis, some commentators have not accepted the validity of the interpretation of these data and continue to suggest that a higher incidence (rather than a higher treatment rate) remains unproven, because of the serious methodological flaws with the research that has been carried out. See Sashidharan (1993) and Sashidharan and Francis (1993) for comprehensive reviews of this. The kind of problems that are focused on include:

- Until the 1991 Census, where a question on ethnic background was asked for the first time, there had been only limited and unreliable data on the size of the ethnic minority populations from which contacts with psychiatric services are drawn, resulting in the possible underestimation of the 'total' population and consequent overestimation of morbidity rates. This problem may also exist for estimates based on the 1991 Census because of its under-enumeration of ethnic minority people (OPCS 1994).
- It is also possible that the number of African-Caribbean people admitted to hospital with a first ever episode of psychosis could be overestimated. Lipsedge (1993) suggests two ways in which this might happen. First, because of the differences in the ways that African-Caribbean and white patients are treated by mental health services (as described below), African-Caribbean patients may be more reluctant to disclose any previous psychiatric treatment. Second, high geographical mobility in this population might lead to records of previous admissions being missed. Both of these would result in studies of contact with psychiatric services for psychosis overestimating the number of African-Caribbean patients with a first admission.
- Given that not all of those with psychosis are admitted to hospital, it is also possible that the data reflect the

differences in the pathways into care for different ethnic groups, which result in African-Caribbean people being more likely than equivalent white people to be admitted. In support of this possibility there is a large body of evidence that suggests that African-Caribbean and other black people are over-represented among patients compulsorily detained in psychiatric hospitals, are more likely to have been in contact with the police or other forensic services prior to admission, and more likely to have been referred to these services by a stranger rather than by a relative or neighbour. This is despite them being both less likely than whites to display evidence of self-harm and no more likely to be aggressive to others prior to admission (Harrison *et al.* 1989; Rogers 1990; McKenzie *et al.* 1995; Davies *et al.* 1996).

● It is also possible that differences in the attitudes of health care workers to different ethnic groups and difficulties in the diagnosis of schizophrenia may be involved. For example, McKenzie *et al.* (1995) showed that African-Caribbean people with psychosis were less likely than equivalent whites to have received psychotherapy or antidepressants; Harrison *et al.* (1989) showed that although African-Caribbean people were no more likely to have been aggressive at the time of admission, once admitted staff were more likely to perceive them as potentially dangerous both to themselves and to others; and Rogers (1990) showed that psychiatrists were *more* likely than police to consider African-Caribbeans detained under Section 136 as dangerous to others. Coupled with difficulties in diagnosis, these pieces of evidence suggest that the stereotypes that inform the behaviour of health care workers may make them more likely to diagnose African-Caribbean people as psychotic.

Interestingly, very similar criticisms have been made of epidemiological work showing higher rates of psychosis among black Americans in the United States (Adebimpe 1994). Taken together, these comments suggested that there are a variety of potential problems with existing work and, consequently, that there must remain some doubt about the higher rates of psychosis reported among the African-Caribbean group.

It is equally possible that the reported differences between white and South Asian groups and the inconsistencies found in these could, as for the African-Caribbean group, be a result of the methodological limitations of studies in this area. In addition to the difficulties of relying on treatment data, outlined above, the lower rates of mental illness among South Asian people could reflect language and communication difficulties, or a general reluctance among South Asian people to consult with doctors over mental health problems. More fundamentally, they may reflect a difference in the symptomatic experience of South Asian people with a mental illness compared with white people. In particular, it has been suggested that South Asian people may experience particular 'culture-bound' syndromes, that is a cluster of symptoms which is restricted to a particular culture, such as sinking heart (Krause 1989), and consequently not be identified as mentally ill.

More fundamentally, the reliance of psychiatric research on the identification of clusters of symptoms that reflect an underlying disease, and the potentially different idioms for expressing mental distress in different cultures, allow for what Kleinman (1987) describes as a 'category fallacy'. He argues that the use for research or treatment in a particular culture of a category of illness that was developed in another cultural group, may fail to identify many to whom it can apply, because it lacks coherence in that culture. The idioms of mental distress in the researched group are simply different from those used in the research tool. So, Kleinman (1987) points out the obvious fallacy in attempting to identify the prevalence of 'semen loss' or 'soul loss' in white Western groups. This may, of course, equally be the case for instruments designed to detect Western expressions of mental distress when applied to other cultures. Indeed, Jadhav (1996) has been able to describe the historical and regional development of 'Western depression', leading him to suggest that this apparently universal disorder is culturally specific.

There has only been limited empirical work in this area so there is only limited evidence to support this position. In one example, Fenton and Sadiq-Sangster (1996) identified an expression of distress that they described, using their respondents' words, as 'thinking too much in my heart'. While they found that this correlated strongly with the expression of most of the standard Western symptoms of depression, they were also able to show that some of these standard symptoms were not present (those relating to a loss of meaning in life and self-worth), suggesting that at least the form that the disease took was different. They also pointed out that 'thinking too much in my heart' was not only a symptom as such, but a core experience of the illness, raising the possibility that there were more fundamental differences between this illness and depression.

In addition to the problems with using treatment statistics and with conducting cross-cultural research into mental health, a number of other methodological problems restrict the confidence with which we can interpret data on ethnic differences in mental health. Many studies use country of birth as a surrogate for ethnicity, because they either use pre-1991 Census data to calculate the denominator (e.g. Cochrane and Bal's (1989) analysis of hospital admissions) or they use mortality data, which record country of birth but not ethnicity (e.g. Raleigh (1996) analysis of death by suicide).

Survey data on the relationship between ethnicity and mental health, such as those provided by the FNS, present a number of additional problems. First, many surveys of ethnic minority people are carried out in particular locations and consequently have restricted generalizability beyond that geographical context (e.g. Bhugra *et al.* 1997). Second, many studies that claim to be nationally representative often only cover areas with large ethnic minority populations, so ethnic minority people living in predominantly white areas are not included. Third, survey data inevitably suffer from a non-response problem, where some of those who are identified for inclusion in the survey refuse to co-operate and such refusal may be related to the condition under study. Fourth, the condition under study might be sufficiently rare in the community and be sufficiently hard to detect (as, for example, in the case of psychotic disorders) as to require both large samples and complicated procedures for estimating prevalence, making the estimate imprecise (i.e. leaving large standard errors).

It is worth raising a final problem with much of the data used to examine ethnic differences in mental health, which is the failure to include explanatory variables for observed relationships.

The range of potential explanations for observed associations between ethnic background and mental health are described in the next section, but very often no attempt is made to assess them in studies, which typically simply document relative rates for ethnic minority groups compared with the white 'norm'. This, as one of us has argued at some length elsewhere (Nazroo 1998; see also Sheldon and Parker 1992), simply allows both the author and reader of reports to make assumptions about the nature of the relationship, commonly based on stereotypes about the cultural or genetic attributes of the ethnic minority groups under study.

Explaining key findings and contradictions

The kind of explanations considered for ethnic differences in mental health are similar to those considered for other ethnic inequalities in health in the epidemiological literature described by Dyson and Smaje (Chapter 2, this volume).

Migration

First, different rates of mental health across migrant and non-migrant groups could be a consequence of factors related to the actual process of migration. Social selection into a migrant group could have favoured those with a higher or lower risk of developing illness, or the stresses associated with migration might have increased risks. There is evidence to both support and counter these suggestions. In the case of the apparently higher rates of schizophrenia among African-Caribbeans in Britain, investigations of the rates of schizophrenia in Jamaica and Trinidad suggest that they are much lower than those for African-Caribbean people in Britain and, in fact, similar to those of the white population of Britain (Hickling 1991; Hickling and Rodgers-Johnson 1995; Bhugra *et al.* 1996). This would suggest that the higher rates are either a consequence of factors related to the migration process, or of the circumstances surrounding the lives of ethnic minority people in Britain.

However, if the higher rates were a consequence of stress around migration, we would expect other migrant groups also to have higher rates of mental illness. As described earlier, evidence here is contradictory. On the whole studies have suggested that other migrants to Britain, in particular South Asian people, do not have similarly raised rates (Cochrane and Bal 1989), although, as described earlier, King *et al.* (1994) strongly came to the conclusion that the risk of schizophrenia was markedly higher in all migrant groups (including white migrant groups). In addition, if the higher rates of schizophrenia among African-Caribbeans were a consequence of selection into a migrant group or the stresses associated with migration, one would expect the rates for those born in Britain to begin to approximate those of the white population. However, as described above, studies have suggested that rates of schizophrenia for African-Caribbean people born in Britain are even higher than for those who migrated (McGovern and Cope 1987; Harrison *et al.* 1988), suggesting that factors relating directly to the process of migration may not be involved, although these data (like most work in this area) are dependent on a very small number of identified cases.

Genetic differences

As with all work on ethnicity and health, there has been discussion of the possibility that differences may be a consequence of a genetic factor that correlates with ethnic background, but little supporting evidence has been marshalled. Evidence suggests large differences in risk within ethnic categories, implying that any genetic basis for mental illness does not correlate closely with ethnic background. For example, the evidence on schizophrenia cited in the previous section, which shows that there are important differences between African-Caribbean people who stayed in Jamaica or Trinidad (who do not have raised rates), those who migrated to Britain (who appear to have raised rates), and those who were born in Britain (who appear to have markedly raised rates), suggests that the higher rates cannot be straightforward consequence of ethnic differences in genetic risk.

Culture

Not surprisingly, most research that has focused on cultural explanations for ethnic differences in mental health has based the cultural argument on speculative and stereotyped characterizations of the cultures of ethnic minority groups, which do not acknowledge the dynamic nature of culture (Ahmad 1996a).

The use of cultural explanations for differences in risk of mental illness between whites and South Asians is instructive. Here stereotyped notions of South Asian communities have been mobilized in markedly different ways to explain both low and high rates of illness. So, in language that is reminiscent of (though it predates its recent popularity in the health inequalities field) the concept of social capital, it has been suggested that the overall lower rates of mental illness among South Asian people could be a consequence of a strong and protective Asian culture, which provides extended and strong communities with protective social support networks (Cochrane and Bal 1989). In contrast, in the attempt to explain the high mortality rates of suicide among young women born in South Asia, close and extended South Asian communities are portrayed as demanding, constraining and conflictual, and as contributing to the higher suicide rates rather than supportive and cohesive (Raleigh and Balarajan 1992).

Of course, a closer examination shows that such stereotypes may not hold. For example, despite the focus on patriarchal South Asian families, there are great similarities between the motives of white and South Asian patients for their suicidal actions. For example, in one study of attempted suicide, Handy *et al.* (1991) say that arguments with parents were a common factor for both white and Asian children, and in another study of attempted suicide Merrill and Owens' examples of: restrictive Asian customs (e.g. not allowing them to go out at night, mix with boys, or take further education) (1986: 709) are not greatly different from what one might find in a dispute between a young white woman and her parents. Indeed, a study of coroners' reports on actual suicides in London found that only one third of the twelve South Asian women who had committed suicide had 'family conflict' cited among the reasons for the suicide, and only by stretching the imagination could these be considered as specific to South Asian cultures (Karmi *et al.* 1994).

Racism and socio-economic position

Different rates in mental health across different ethnic groups might be a consequence of the different forms of discrimination and racism that ethnic minority people face in Britain. This could be a direct result of the experience of discrimination and harassment, or a result of the social disadvantages that racism leads to. Recent evidence has described both the nature and extent of the harassment ethnic minority people are subjected to (Virdee 1995, 1997), and it would not be surprising if the multiple victimization that some are subjected to led to mental distress.

Alternatively, the exclusionary effects of racism might also lead to ethnic differences in mental health as a result of the consequent poorer circumstances of ethnic minority groups. So, it would also not be surprising if the poor, run down, inner city environments and poor housing in which many ethnic minority people live, and their poorer employment prospects and standards of living (Modood *et al.* 1997), led to greater mental distress (King *et al.* 1994). As elsewhere in the ethnicity and health field (Sheldon and Parker 1992), there has been considerable criticism of the failure to take into account explanatory variables related to social disadvantage in research that links ethnicity to poor mental health, as there is a strong possibility that these underlie the relationship (Sashidharan 1993; Sashidharan and Francis 1993). These authors suggest that ignoring the possibility that the relationship between ethnicity and health is a consequence of social disadvantage allows the theoretical alignment of psychiatric disorder with an essentialized ethnic difference. Psychiatric disorder becomes one of the essentialized attributes of certain ethnic minority groups and this leads to the suggestion that psychiatric disorder is a consequence of some inherent and stable characteristic of certain ethnic minority groups. This in turn leads to the cultural and biological heritage of those groups becoming medicalized, enabling the process of racialization to occur. In support of the socio-economic argument, findings from the FNS do suggest that there is a marked socio-economic patterning of risk of mental disorder within all of the ethnic groups covered, and that this patterning contributed to differences across groups (Nazroo 1997b).

Mental health services

In addition to considering the impact of racism on health, either direct or through consequent adverse socio-economic circumstances (Nazroo 1998), it is also important to explore and address how such social disadvantage influences ethnic minority patients' experiences of and uptake of mental health services and the implications of this for practice.

Generally, regardless of their ethnic background people with mental health problems are critical of the services they receive (Audit Commission 1994a; King's Fund 1998; Sainsburys Centre for Mental Health 1998a, 1998b). Common criticisms revolve around the fact that the mainstay of services are acute hospital units which are poorly staffed, leading to a lack of therapeutic intervention and a lack of information giving from staff. Not surprisingly, this has lead to suggestions that services could be improved by providing more 24-hour support in the community.

Several more specific issues have been raised when the mental health care needs of ethnic minority people have been considered (Sainsburys Centre for Mental Health 1998a; King's Fund 1998). Common criticisms have included a feeling of not being listened to and a general feeling of cultural insensitivity shown by healthare staff. Such cultural insensitivity is likely to be reflected in the stereotypes used by healthcare workers when dealing with ethnic minority people, stereotypes such as African-Caribbean people being 'Big, Black and dangerous' (Webbe 1998), which might also be reflected in the greater likelihood of psychiatrists compared with police to perceive African-Caribbean patients detained under Section 136 as dangerous (Rogers 1990). And these stereotypes are, because of the lack of teaching on cultural diversity during, for example, nurse education (Gerrish et al. 1996; Webbe 1998), rarely formally challenged and may be deeply rooted in the clinical practice of healthcare workers. For example, one study has suggested that despite South Asian patients consulting their GPs with mental health problems, their symptoms often went undiagnosed (Commander *et al.* 1997), perhaps because of the cross-cultural limits of Western diagnostic categories (Kleinman 1987; Jadhav 1996). And the FNS found that Caribbean people who had scored on a depression inventory were far less likely than white people to be receiving treatment despite being as likely to have contacted their GP (Nazroo 1997b).

Ethnic minority users of mental health services have also indicated that they are suspicious of statutory mental health services and their suspicion appears to be based on previous negative experiences. Worryingly some users have said that they are fearful of dying in hospital as a result of the over use of medication and the aggressive restraining techniques employed by staff (Sainsburys Centre for Mental Health 1998a). We have already indicated that there is some wider evidence to support such suspicions. African-Caribbean patients are more likely to be compulsorily admitted to hospital despite not being more likely to be a danger to themselves or others (Harrison *et al.* 1989; Rogers 1990; McKenzie *et al.* 1995; Davies *et al.* 1996). Similarly, African-Caribbean patients with a diagnosis of psychosis remain in acute hospital care longer than white patients and have more frequent outpatient follow-up contacts, despite having fewer negative symptoms (Takei *et al.* 1998). Yet, despite this over-representation in the acute sector, when discharged into the community it seems that African-Caribbean patients receive inadequate support from community mental health teams (Audit Commission 1994a).

Although these problems have been repeatedly acknowledged (e.g. Mental Health Foundation 1995; King's Fund 1998), little action appears to have followed. It seems that unless the root causes of these problems are tackled, they will continue to surface and be acknowledged in reports and policy documents, but fail to be addressed. Nevertheless, such reports have included several recommendations for change, including involving service users and voluntary groups in planning future service provision. It is suggested that more joint working between voluntary and statutory agencies would provide more flexible community based services and help purchasers and providers to ensure that staff and services provide culturally diverse services (King's Fund 1998). It certainly seems that the depth of experience in the voluntary sector could be a valuable resource for both the planning of statutory services and the development of individual practitioners. And there is some evidence that ethnic minority service users and voluntary groups can be effectively involved in planning mental health service provision. For example, in Manchester an African-Caribbean mental health project has been established to provide an outreach and advocacy service using a multi-disciplinary team approach (Mental Health Foundation 1995). Also, at Lewisham and Guy's Mental Health NHS Trust, service users and voluntary groups were involved in the development of a new intensive care unit at a local hospital, an involvement that included the recruitment of staff and policy formation (Sainsburys Centre for Mental Health 1998b). These examples of good practice are built upon a model of partnership between the acute hospital setting, community care teams, voluntary organizations, and patients and their carers. But, of course, as with changes in other sectors (Ahmad 1993), many of these initiatives have only evolved as a result of pressure from voluntary groups, or patients and their carers themselves. Also most of these services tend to be located in areas with high concentrations of ethnic minority people, which does little to address the problems faced by ethnic minority people who live in other areas of the country, where factors such as a lack of cultural awareness and assumptions about behaviour may play a greater role in aggravating poor service provision (Audit Commission 1994a).

Another recurring recommendation made by policy makers, service users and voluntary groups is that healthcare professionals should receive training and education about cultural diversity. However, for this to be effective requires a careful review of what we actually mean by cultural diversity along with a careful consideration of how to educate practitioners to deal with the issues involved. Certainly, many attempts to address cultural diversity in educational materials have failed or, worse still, been based on stereotypical images of ethnic minority groups. Examples of this can be seen in a number of mental health nursing textbooks from the United States, which offer lists of expected behaviours from specific ethnic groups, and papers in medical journals and textbooks in which reference to voodoo and other 'cultural practices' are discussed in relation to mental illness (e.g. Dein 1997). These types of educational resources can only serve to reinforce the negative and inappropriate attitudes and behaviours of some healthcare professionals. Examples of providing culturally sensitive education to healthcare professionals in the mental health field appear to be sparse, with most of the literature relating to this subject going no further than recommending the implementation of training and education (e.g. Gerrish *et al.* 1996; King's Fund 1998; Webbe 1998). This clearly needs to be addressed urgently, with the inclusion in all health professionals' curricula of teaching on the concepts of ethnicity and identity, along with cultural competency training (learning the principles and skills that enable the trainee to discover the relevant cultural dimensions of the populations they serve (Bhopal and White 1993)), and patient advocacy training.

Of course, we should remain aware of the possibility that racism lies at the route of the problems that we have been outlining (Ahmad 1993; Smaje 1995a; Burr and Chapman 1998). This suggests the need for a strengthening of anti-discrimination legislation and anti-discrimination policies and practices in health care settings. However, history has shown that legislation and policies to overcome discrimination may not have a great impact on practice. For example, despite the presence of equal opportunities policies and the 1976 Race Relations Act, in the specific arena of healthcare in England ethnic minority people have been discriminated against when applying for medical school places (McManus *et al.* 1995) and ethnic minority nurses working in the NHS have a slower career progression than their white equivalents (Beishon *et al.* 1995).

Processes of ethnic identification and racism

This review suggests that many basic questions concerning the relationship between ethnicity and mental health remain unanswered. There remains a question of whether the use of Western psychiatric instruments for the cross-cultural measurement of psychiatric disorder is valid and produces a genuine reflection of the differences between different ethnic groups (Kleinman 1987; Littlewood 1992; Jadhav 1996). This has been raised particularly in relation to the low detection and treatment rates for depressive disorders among South Asians, but may apply to other disorders and other ethnic minority groups. It is also likely that treatment-based statistics do not accurately reflect the experiences of the populations from which those in treatment are drawn.

Perhaps, as others have pointed out (Sashidharan and Francis 1993), the most important conclusion to draw is that it is vital to avoid essentializing ethnic differences in mental health (i.e. reducing them to stereotyped notions of fixed cultural or biological difference). There is a need to explore the factors associated with ethnicity that may explain any relationship between ethnicity and mental health, such as the various forms of social disadvantage faced by ethnic minority people. And it remains important to explore how racism and the social disadvantages that this leads to structure the experiences of ethnic minority people when they come into contact with mental health services.

Despite this, the focus on biological explanations for mental illness continues in both the USA and the UK (Munro 1999). And media fuelled public concerns about mental illness appear to be influencing current policy making (Munro 1999). This has implications for the future role of mental health nursing, with a risk of a return to a more coercive role in care delivery, such as enforcing treatment orders. This, coupled with racism, presents major difficulties for those working in this clinical speciality. The challenge for mental health nurses is to consider these issues when delivering care that encompasses the individual in their social context.

Although throughout we have emphasized the central role of racism and consequent socio-economic disadvantage, the wider sociological literature on ethnicity and 'race' has also placed great importance on the notion of ethnic identity, which reflects self-identification with cultural traditions that provide both meaning and boundaries between groups. So, although some argue that socio-economic disadvantage might contribute to ethnic inequalities in health and access to health services, it is suggested that there remains a cultural component to ethnicity that could play a major defining role (Smaje 1996).

Not surprisingly, the sociological focus on ethnicity as identity has mirrored the anti-essentialism found in work on identity more generally (Modood 1998). So, although ethnicity is considered to reflect identification with sets of shared values, beliefs, customs and lifestyles, it has to be understood dynamically, as an active social process (Smaje 1996). In particular, the influence of the culture of individuals and groups on their health has to be properly contextualized. The emphasis is on *agency*, the construction of identity and how this depends on wider contexts, personal biographies and factors such as gender and class (Ahmad 1996a).

Of course, as with any attempt to provide a sociological understanding, and as our discussion of racism implies, it is also important to consider ethnicity as *structure*. Here Miles' (1989) portrayal of racism as central to an understanding of ethnic or 'race' relations is of great use. When discussing the emergence of ethnic or 'race' categories within a society Miles emphasizes how ethnic difference can be essentialised as a product of 'nature' and how this becomes a justification for exclusionary and discriminatory treatment (Miles 1996). This reminds us that a core component of ethnic relations involves the categorization of the Other and the exclusion of the Other.

Miles' comments are a reminder that ethnic identity is assigned as well as adopted (and assigned on the basis of power relations). So, ethnicity needs to be examined as both agency (a contextualized culture) and structure (racism and socio-economic disadvantage) when considering ethnic inequalities in mental health.

Mental health and nursing practice

Nurses have a clear role to play as part of the mental health care team in working closely with users, their carers and voluntary organizations to provide services which are user-friendly, appropriately funded and culturally and socially accessible (Bhugra and Bahl 1999). There has been very little research which specifically examines the delivery of nursing care to minority ethnic groups in mental health settings. Narayanasamy (1999) has suggested some practical ways in which a positive nurse/client relationship might be established, involving negotiation and compromise, the establishment of respect and rapport and the promotion of a sense of cultural safety. Nurses urgently need to develop a research agenda to inform their clinical practice and develop new ways of working to support and communicate effectively with minority ethnic users. Within the existing evidence base, nurses can usefully familiarize themselves with information on the wider context of the relationship between ethnicity and mental illness, examine research on pathways to mental health care and the literature on how minority ethnic people experience psychiatry. They can also be closely involved in actively making contact with communities and developing an understanding of users' perspectives and criticisms of current service provision. Several of the contributors to Bhugra and Bahl (1999) discuss ways in which mental health professionals in a variety of primary care and acute settings can promote good clinical practice, create an atmosphere of understanding and build confidence within their users from minority ethnic groups. Improving the management of mental illness in clinical practice is vital, but community nurses in particular are well placed to become involved in preventative strategies based on public health models, working with communities in schools and places of work.

Conclusion

This chapter has outlined some reasons for the controversial nature of the field of mental health and minority ethnic groups. It examined key findings in the areas of psychotic illness, depression and suicide. Using contact with mental health services as a measure of levels of mental illness may reflect the stereotypes health professionals hold of, say, African-Caribbean patients, rather than levels of illness. Different ways in which mental illness may find cultural expression may mean mental illness in other ethnic groups is not identified. The association between ethnicity and rates of mental illness is not itself an explanation of that illness and does not in itself help a nurse with her care.

The chapter has also reviewed possible explanations of inequalities in mental health among different ethnic groups.

Since British-born ethnic minorities have higher rates of mental illness than migrants to Britain who in turn have higher rates than those who remain in their country of origin, this suggests that neither genetics nor migration are strong explanations of any differences. Culture has been misused as a possible explanation, and allegedly 'cultural' reasons for suicide often amount to issues of generation or family conflict common to all ethnic groups. However, racism and socio-economic disadvantage may underlie the relationship between ethnicity and mental illness.

The mental health services themselves may compound inequalities in mental health to the extent that the treatment of African-Caribbeans is over-aggressive and those of South Asian descent are under-identified and under-referred for treatment. Examples of good practice are rare, but usually involve joint working with ethnic minority service users.

We have suggested that mental health nurses working with patients from minority ethnic groups need to bear in mind lessons from both the sociological concepts of agency and of structure. People's experience and expression of mental illness is bound up in the processes of actively constructing their own identities, which may involve elements of life history, age and gender as well as ethnicity. Patterns of racism and socio-economic disadvantage facing minority ethnic groups may provoke mental illnesses in ways we still need to explore. Racism and socio-economic disadvantage may also structure the experiences of minority ethnic groups when and if they are in contact with mental health services.

Finally, ways forward in practice include working with carers and voluntary organizations; learning to negotiate care with the client; researching local needs and experiences of the service provided and engaging in preventative strategies based on public health models.

4 Ethnic monitoring and nursing

Mark R D Johnson

Introduction

Since April 1996, the NHS has expected all hospital trusts to record, and provide as part of the 'contract minimum data set' to purchasers, data relating to the ethnic origins of all 'admitted patients'. This includes those who are admitted to hospital for any form of treatment, as well as day cases that come under their care. The circular authorizing this process (NHS Executive EL(94)77) was the product of considerable discussion and prior testing, and led to considerable controversy at the time (Johnson and Gill 1995; Ranger 1994). Since then, there has been a steady growth in the collection of the data, although rather less signs of its use. Similar learning pains have been experienced in the criminal justice system (Fitzgerald and Sibbitt 1997). More recently, the NHS has supported development of ethnic monitoring procedures in primary care (Pringle and Rothera 1996), and several 'pilot sites', in West London (Brent and Harrow), the West Midlands, and Liverpool, have been training staff so that the data may be collected by staff working in GP surgeries. Nurses entering practice now, may therefore expect to come across this activity in their everyday work. They need to know both about the implementation of ethnic monitoring, and about its possible value to their own clinical practice.

This chapter introduces the concepts of ethnic record keeping and ethnic monitoring, and some of the frequently asked questions about their practice. It describes the value of the data and procedures to the practice of nursing, and some of the problems encountered. In particular, it considers arguments for and against ethnic monitoring, and the categories used in data collection. In the process, it explores some of the concepts of ethnicity, and discusses the relevance of this in practice. It shows links to the uses and implementation of ethnic monitoring in other sectors of public service provision, and the use made there of such data, and discusses some of the issues that arise in joint agency working.

What is ethnic monitoring?

Simply stated, it would seem that ethnic monitoring is the process of asking people about their ethnic origins – the ethnic group to which they belong – and recording that information in the databases which all agencies, including hospitals and the NHS, necessarily keep for their own use. This, however, leaves certain questions unanswered: what is ethnic origin: is it different from 'ethnic group', and how can we tell what a person's ethnic group is? How should it be entered in the records? How useful is the information to the practitioner, and what can the nurse or other person say when asked why the information is being collected? What happens if someone refuses to give this information? Is it legal to ask about 'race' or is this in fact discrimination?

It will be immediately obvious to nurses and those caring for people that not all their clients are the same – and that some of these differences have implications for the provision of services. Very few people in the health and caring services and other public sectors would like to think that they discriminated against their users, on grounds of their 'race', religion or national origins. However, in 1999 the Macpherson Inquiry into the death of Stephen Lawrence, a young black man from South London, was in no doubt that the Metropolitan Police had shown signs of 'institutional racism' (Macpherson 1999). By this, they meant unintentional discrimination against people whose cultures and origins had not been considered when services had been set up. The Government pledged itself to eliminate this problem, both within the criminal justice system, and in the health service and other public services. Ethnic monitoring – making explicit these differences and taking account of them in monitoring and planning services, is part of the necessary solution.

General policy is not however necessarily neutral. If policy favours one language, one religion or (more generally) one view, or even imposes them on all the people, that policy is general but not neutral . . .

To develop . . . policies when they are aimed partly or wholly at ethnically defined categories in society, it is essential to gather reliable information about the composition of that multi-ethnic society. (Vermeulen 1997: 10–12)

Bureaucracies thrive on collection of information, but the statement of a policy, and the recording of some data, are not sufficient evidence of a change in the way the organisation operates! Ethnic monitoring is one of several ways that the administration can examine service up-take and outcomes. The information thus gained then must be related to some objectives and standards which have been set as part of a policy for the allocation of resources and expected outcomes (Connelly 1988). Record keeping without monitoring is a pointless exercise, and wasteful of resources. If information is collected and nothing is done to consider the implications of what it shows, it becomes a redundant exercise. Staff will resent making the effort to collect information, and minority communities will question why the data are being collected. This can lead to future mistrust of other well-meant initiatives, and that will render more difficult the job of the nurse who is providing care.

Thus while ethnic record keeping is *necessary* if monitoring is to take place it is not *sufficient*. Ethnic monitoring is a *process* whereby information about the relevant aspects of people's ethnic origins is collected, recorded, and used to establish patterns, which can be compared with other information about their relationship with society and 'need'. In the best cases, this information is used to set targets and establish policies which will overcome disadvantage and lead to improvements in service delivery and the material circumstances of the members of minorities. At the very least, it can be used to establish the facts and make a case for such changes to be attempted.

In some services, furthermore, a direct functional value can be adduced for the maintenance of ethnic monitoring and related information systems. There is clearly a direct link between the proportion of Muslims in a community and the likely demand for halal food, and other facilities to enable patients to practice their Islamic faith. Sheldon and Parker (1992), Ahmad and Sheldon (1993) and Bradby (1995) all argue that we should ask directly about food choices, rather than assuming that 'ethnic group' categories will enable us to predict these. However, we shall return to this question. There are, for example, other reasons for finding out about peoples' origins. Certain diseases (while not *exclusively* confined to certain minorities) are much more commonly encountered in certain minority groups (see Chapter 7). However, European people from Sweden are five times more likely than the Dutch to carry the 'Factor V Leiden' gene which can raise their risk of (potentially fatal) deep vein thrombosis (Vandenbroucke *et al.* 1996). While some data on birthplace may be available from the census, this does not help with religious orientations, nor can census data give information about changing population profiles or the arrival in an area of refugees from a particular group after the census has taken place. As Europe becomes increasingly a society of settled migrants, with third and fourth generations born in countries to which their grandparents may have moved inheriting the risk of diseases less common among people usually described as 'native born', this sort of question will become more, rather than less, urgent. Further, inefficiencies can be exposed through ethnic monitoring, as well as new opportunities to deliver service or to recruit 'customers' and thereby justify expenditure. 'Minority' clients, it should be remembered, have 'majority' needs as well.

What should be recorded for the monitoring?

There are many ways of defining an 'ethnic minority' (Pringle *et al.* 1997). Equally, some people feel it very hard to ask about such differences – it may seem to be rather personal or sensitive information, although nurses and other health workers have become used to asking very personal questions about health in the course of their work! Frequently one characteristic or another is used as a proxy for the difference: this may provide a solution to the needs of the would-be monitor of the needs and experiences of service clients, but that is not certain. The crucial issue is that any categorization used is relevant to the delivery of a service and recognition of a 'client's' need.

> The trouble with using nationality, birthplace, ethnic origin or language spoken at home as indicators of ethnic categories is that this implicitly assumes that such criteria all refer to the same clear-cut entities ... It is more effective to use different criteria to pursue different policy objectives ... (Vermeulen 1997: 12)

It will be clear from the discussion so far that 'ethnic monitoring' requires the identification of individuals as belonging to one or more groups, defined in terms of culture and origin. However, were it nothing more than this, it would be no more than the sort of casual categorization that can lead to discrimination and harm based on stereotype (Ahmad 1999). To be effective and useful, ethnic monitoring must rely upon the individual concerned being given the opportunity to define their identity in terms that are meaningful to them – and hence, which reveal something about them which is of value to the care-giver. This may mean looking for differences where they are not expected – including differences among the 'white majority' population that cannot be inferred from skin colour and appearance. It is apparent from this that the nurse, or any other person seeking to deliver a service, must first consider what factors are relevant to their work and the ways in which 'ethnic' differences affect the ways in which people need or use their service.

We may start to consider certain specific issues around which groups may be differentiated, and the implications this has. Ethnic monitoring requires careful consideration of the characteristics which are of most relevance to the service. It may be that the 'ethnic group' labels such as those used in the UK 1991 Census – 'Black-Caribbean', 'Asian-Pakistani' and so on, are sufficient to identify the existence of discrimination on broad, racialized grounds. These terms are, for many, what is understood by the phrase 'ethnicity'. For many purposes, this will be enough, at least to alert policy makers to the need to investigate matters more closely. However, for planning services and allocating resources, as suggested above, more detailed information is likely to be needed, and the Office for National Statistics has agreed that the 2001 Census should ask new questions.

While some categories such as 'Pakistani' may be associated fairly closely with particular cultural characteristics such as language (Urdu), religion (Muslim) and perhaps certain aspects of lifestyle, it is dangerous to assume that this will always be the case – the language and social preferences of Pathan (Pushto-speaking) people from the north-west of Pakistan are quite distinct from those who sometimes describe themselves as Kashmiris or Pakistani Punjabis from the north-east of the same state. Their children too may ascribe different labels to themselves. However, when numbers are small, the 'ideal' solution of allowing everyone to self-identify their preferred label may lead to inaction on the basis that there are too many differences to plan for. In such cases, it is best to offer broad categories ('Asian', 'African-Caribbean') to establish overall patterns, supplemented by additional questions about issues such as language, religion and diet which may require the provision of specific services in order to meet genuine personal needs. Obviously, these questions also need to be asked of those who appear to be 'white' – who will also belong to religious, cultural and possibly linguistic groups whose needs must be taken account of.

One of the least threatening and most commonly used identifiers, is that of 'mother tongue' or 'language most commonly used in the home' – which can be seen to relate directly to the needs of the client. Increasingly, hospitals and community health trusts employ, or have access to, an interpreter service. Unless language is asked about, and recorded, managers may have no idea of the need for this service. Increasing numbers of refugees, and older people who settled in Britain after the Second World War (from India, Italy and Poland, among other places), need such help. Clearly, it would be best if the information was recorded the first time the person used the health services (such as at the GP), and then their possible need for an interpreter could follow them in referral letters: this seldom happens. At least, if the records are kept and used properly, it can be seen that there is a need! At the same time, however, asking may raise expectations – which in the way of justice and efficiency, should be met (See Chapter 6, this volume).

There is some evidence that appointments may be wasted (through non-attendance: 'DNA') because of the failure to provide an interpreter – or because appointment letters are sent out in English when they cannot be read (Audit Commission 1994b; Leman 1997). Language, then, should be at least one of the items of information included in ethnic monitoring. Most of the common Asian languages use a distinctive script, Urdu using a form of Arabic, Punjabi as spoken by Sikhs the Gurmukhi script, and so on. If necessary, a simple card with a short phrase in the language could be offered to patients, who could indicate which was theirs – even if they were generally unable to read the script. This could also be linked to a reference number, avoiding problems for staff who are unfamiliar with the names of all the possible languages and dialects that may be found. A recent survey of London, for example, came up with more than 150 different languages being spoken in its schools – and when refugees come, they may bring new languages.

Religion can play an important part in caring for people in distress. The role of hospital chaplains is well established, for example, and it is very important to observe the correct procedures in respect of the care of the dying and the treatment of bodies after death. Indeed, most hospital records do have a space for religion, although it is not always filled in, and the 'hospital chaplain' (usually Anglican) often visits everyone who comes in to the wards. The introduction of the 'Patients Charter', with 'Charter Standard 1' which referred explicitly to respect for religion and culture, provided an incentive for many trusts to introduce or upgrade their recording of religion. Indeed, I found many white long-term residents of towns such as Coventry and Bedford welcomed the opportunity to explain that they were Irish and Catholic, or Ukrainian and Orthodox Christians, when I was working with the health trusts to develop ethnic monitoring and language support services. To them, this was an important part of their identity, and it helped them to feel that this might now be understood and taken into account.

The most common indicator of difference, or the size of 'minority' populations, in census data and other official records, is birthplace. This information is recorded on most identity documents, and is used to analyse data such as that collected on death certificates. Unfortunately, it provides a poor indicator of cultural or 'ethnic' origin: many well-known British figures were born in parts of the former British Empire, and have little in common with the more traditional populations of those places! Equally, it is now true that more than half of the 'minority' ethnic population of Britain which can trace its parents' or grandparents' origins to India, Africa and the Caribbean was actually itself born in Britain. In terms of ethnic monitoring, birthplace data are of no value whatsoever, even if still used in some epidemiological studies.

Nationality is probably one of the most problematic categories. Too often the notion of ethnic 'origin' is described as nationality and confused with that of citizenship – that is, passport. Indeed, in some of the 'newer' states of Europe such as Lithuania, it is possible to have one's ethnic origin recorded on the national passport. To others, the notion of nationality implies a homogenous category, and 'foreigners' may have lesser protection under the law. In ethnic monitoring, it is essential not to confuse the idea of identity with the question of the rights of the citizen to state-funded services. Visitors to Britain have certain rights, but may be charged for any non-emergency treatment: to ask British citizens for their passports is offensive and may be discriminatory (Gordon and Newnham 1985).

Why monitor?

Several reasons for the introduction of monitoring have been at least implicitly described already, including those of organizational efficiency, allocation of resources, and the making explicit of the patterns of use of a service. There may also be legal reasons – it may, for example, be necessary to demonstrate explicitly that one is not discriminating, and this can only be done by the production of data from monitoring exercises. Formal investigations conducted by the Commission for Racial Equality frequently end by serving a legal 'enforcement notice' requiring the agency to set up systems of ethnic monitoring and to produce periodic reports relating to their progress.

However, it has to be admitted that there have been voices raised in opposition to the introduction of monitoring. Most frequently, it has been suggested that by monitoring and thus drawing attention to difference, one is somehow discriminating. Resistance to keeping 'ethnic group' data often refers to the misuse of racially categorized records and to issues of civil liberty. Most evidently perhaps, and quite understandably, such accounts refer to the Holocaust and the use made of bureaucratic files by the Nazis to identify Jewish individuals and families. It is not surprising that sensitivity remains over this particular issue, although it may be argued that the identification of the majority of ethnic minorities does not require such bureaucratic assistance. Members of most minorities are aware just how easily they can be identified and discriminated against, without recourse to documentation. In some cases opposition is founded upon a belief in the value of a 'colour-blind' approach. The chief objection to the use of ethnic monitoring, however, has often come from those who see it as a covert means of giving preferential treatment to a particular group. It should be clear that neither of these two (directly opposing) views is accurate!

Most objections have been justified on administrative or practical grounds or made by 'gatekeepers' arguing that they were protecting the interests of minorities or the community. It is also argued, as it has been for many years, that there is no intentional discrimination in the system: 'we operate a fair access system, colour blind: none of our staff would discriminate in a racist fashion' is a fair summary of the typical response. This argument, however, seems to have been fairly well confounded by the findings of the Macpherson Inquiry. The argument that only through the introduction of ethnic monitoring can *accidental* (a term many seem to prefer to *institutional*) discrimination be identified and dealt with, is therefore appealing and generally convincing.

There remains one more recent issue, connected with the debate over civil rights and the fear of excessive power becoming concentrated in the hands of the state and others who collect data, particularly using the modern technological power of the computer. That is a general objection to the collection of personal data without the explicit consent of the individual. In 1995 the European Council agreed a Directive which came into force in 1998, that relates to this issue and explicitly mentions 'ethnic origin'. This places significant restriction on the processing of data:

> . . . any processing of personal data must be lawful and fair to the individuals concerned . . . and not excessive in relation to the purposes for which they are processed, whereas such purposes must be explicit and legitimate and must be determined at the time of the collection . . . (European Parliament and Council Directive 95/46/EC: para. 28)

It is however also important to recognize that the ministers and officials involved in drawing up this ruling were aware that such data would be required, and should be used for the public interest. Thus the Directive continues that:

> . . . member states must also be authorised when justified by grounds of important public interest to derogate from the prohibition of processing sensitive categories of data where important reasons of public interest so justify in areas such as *public health and social protection* . . . especially in order to ensure the quality and cost-effectiveness. . . . (emphasis added) (para. 34)

In 'Section III – Special Categories of Processing', particular attention is paid to questions of 'sensitive data', which includes the sorts of information here considered as relevant to ethnic monitoring:

> Paragraph 1: Member states shall prohibit the processing of personal data revealing racial or ethnic origin, political opinions, religious or philosophical beliefs, trade union membership and the processing of data concerning health or sex life. . . .

Again, there are explicit exclusions to this prohibition, which include such situations as those where the 'data subject' has given his (*sic*) explicit consent, or where it is necessary to be able to demonstrate that other national laws such as those relating to discrimination, are not being broken. It may be expected that future attempts to introduce ethnic monitoring may be resisted, perhaps by reference to this Directive. It is equally certain that a good case can be made when it is in the interests of members of minority groups. One of the clearest examples of this is in the health services, as the Directive recognizes.

How should the monitoring be done?

The first stage should be to explain to the client the reason for ethnic monitoring and to establish that the gathering of data on the individual is based on their informed consent. All data on ethnicity should be 'self-assigned' – that is, reflect the individual's own assessment of their identity. They can be assured that there is no 'right answer': those people who have, for example, a dual or 'mixed' heritage, may wish to indicate that fact, or they may prefer to identify with one or other of their parents ancestries. Increasingly, people are asked to indicate their ethnic group when dealing with other service providers, especially those who live in 'social housing' (housing association and local authority accommodation) or use the social services department. This process will therefore become more familiar to them. Indeed, most people who come to hospital have already been asked similar questions before, and have a good idea of what is meant.

In most hospitals and clinics, there will be a 'prompt card' supplied in a variety of languages and scripts. This can be shown to patients who will then be asked to indicate which ethnic group best fits their own description of their identity, or to specify a category if none of those provided seems appropriate. In the case of young children or patients who are for some reason unable to respond for themselves, a close relative should be asked to supply the information (see Chapter 6, this volume, for more discussion of similar situations). Should no such relative be available, it may be necessary for a member of staff to fill in the form/screen using what information may be available (including case notes). In such cases the fact of such action having been taken should be *clearly* identified on the form, and a check made at an early stage with the individual concerned. Appearances can be deceptive – many dark skinned English people are accustomed to being mistaken for Italian, Spanish, or Indian.

Classification of all forms of demographic data is a contentious issue but data collected may be of little value unless it receives some general level of support and is acceptable for comparison with data from other sources. It is therefore normal to utilise the scheme agreed for the 1991 Census of Population by the Office for National Statistics (formerly OPCS), with certain amendments and the addition of questions relating to data required for the delivery of health services. This will ensure that data collected are compatible with that from national sources and the local authority, and not otherwise unduly intrusive. Following the experience of the OPCS in the Census, those wishing to indicate an alternative description of their ethnic origin must be allowed to record this. Classification for analysis purposes can then follow the procedures of OPCS for attribution of additional categories to one of the major groups, to ensure comparability and also to maintain the confidentiality of the individual in published analyses (Aspinall 1995).

Table 4.1 gives the 'supplied' categories used in the 1991 Census and those which, it is expected, will be asked in the 2001 Census. It can be seen that there are some differences, but that most of the 'old' categories can be located in the new ones. Many people had asked for the inclusion of a 'mixed' category, allowing them to recognize both sets of ancestral heritage. For those who actually wrote in 'mixed' in 1991, a special group was created and can be used in analysing the data. The 2001 Census expects to find many more people who wish to describe themselves in this way (since nearly all in 1991 were younger people) and has allowed for this. The ability to self-describe by writing in 'other background', is also made clearer. While the 2001 Census uses the term 'ethnic group', it also makes it clear that this is seen as a matter of 'cultural background'. For Scotland and Northern Ireland, the categories will however be closer to those used in 1991 – except that in Northern Ireland there is an additional group: 'Irish Traveller' – a group which is explicitly recognized by law in the Republic of Ireland.

These categories have been found to be acceptable to most people as describing the main groups to which people feel they belong. It must, however, be clearly understood that the questions are *not* asking about nationality, and neither are they, on their own, sufficient (Hilton 1996). Additional questions are needed, to ask patients/users for their religion (if any) and main or preferred language (and where relevant, if they will need an interpreter). If individual units or services feel it would be useful for their activity to expand upon any of the groups or categories in use, this can be accommodated. Local needs – for example,

Table 4.1 Supplied categories of ethnic group in the GB Census, 1991, and UK Census 2001.

1991 Census	2001 Census
White	White – British White – Irish White – Any other white background (please write in)
(Other . . .)	Mixed – white/black Caribbean Mixed – white/black African Mixed – white/Asian Any other mixed background . . . (please write in)
Black – Caribbean	Black or black British: Caribbean
Black – African	Black or black British: African
Black – other (Please describe)	Black or black British: Any other background: (please write in)
Indian	Asian or Asian British Indian
Pakistani	Asian or Asian British Pakistani
Bangladeshi	Asian or Asian British Bangladeshi
Other groups – Asian	Asian or Asian British Any other background: (please write in)
Chinese	Chinese or other ethnic group Chinese
Any other ethnic group (Please describe)	Chinese or other ethnic group Any other background (please write in)

Note 1: This table does not show the precise layout of the census questions, but shows the groups that most people will tick and the relationship between the categories used in the two census forms.

Note 2: There is no direct comparison between the 1991 'Asian-Other' category and the 2001 'Other-Asian'. For example, Filipinos were included in Asian-Other in 1991, but will be in Other Ethnic Group in 2001.

Source: Office for National Statistics.

to include a category of Vietnamese, or one of the major refugee groups – will mean that each health district may have some extra categories in their scheme. Equally, there will need to be recommended classifications for language and religion, in order to maximize compatibility with other data collected in the area. It is proposed that the 2001 Census will include a question on religion, although it will not ask about languages other than 'Celtic' (Gaelic/Welsh).

Patients who are unwilling for any reason to have their ethnic origin identified, or who decline to offer a category after having received a full explanation (in keeping with the training to be given to all staff likely to find themselves in this situation) should be recorded as 'non-responders'. It is advisable that this category should not be offered as an alternative on the prompt cards. The proportion of such incomplete data records needs to be monitored as an indication of the acceptability and effectiveness of the recording process and the training of staff.

In most places, an explanation of the reasons behind the data collection should accompany the prompt card, and should be summarized on it in written form. The same information could be made available in poster format in public waiting areas. Staff in each trust or agency should be instructed in the purposes of ethnic monitoring and the procedures to be followed locally. They will then be able to assist patients or their relatives in the completion of the form and to understand this policy. They will be able to explain to anyone who needs to know that data from the ethnic monitoring exercise will be stored as part of routine case histories and monitoring data relating to the patient concerned. Access will be subject to the usual limitations, and to the disclosure rules of the Data Protection Act 1984 and other regulations applying to health service data.

In keeping with these regulations, data on the ethnic group classification of the individual should be regarded as wholly confidential and restricted to those directly involved in the care of that individual. However, service providers collecting the data are required to make provision for periodic returns of anonymized aggregated data on the use of their services by ethnic group as part of the normal returns to the health authority and other commissioning bodies. These returns can then be used in the health authority as a basis for service delivery evaluation and monitoring. Units should include an analysis and commentary on their findings in their annual reports, together with action plans if patterns of use are found to deviate from those expected. It is also good practice, although too rarely done, that reports arising from data collection should be published and made generally available to ensure both that patients and public are made aware of the policy and its justifications, and that they may be reassured regarding the use to which the data are put. Where this is done, it also improves the confidence with which the public regards the operation of the general policy making, planning and information systems of the trust or authority. Indeed, examples can be found of this happening not only in Britain, but also in other countries where multicultural-ism and cultural safety in nursing have become accepted as the standard best practice (McAvoy *et al.* 1994; Barclay *et al.* 1993). Viewed in this way, ethnic monitoring is not just a special pro-cedure, but an integral part of the processes of clinical audit and performance management.

Conclusion

Ethnic monitoring is a fairly new, and still developing tool which has value for both 'management by information' approaches and the implementation of equal opportunity policies. It provides new ways of examining the effectiveness and quality of service provision and employment practice, taking into account all the different elements of personal identity encompassed by the concept of 'ethnicity'. These include religion, language, and cul-tural background, all of which have clinical relevance for com-munication and care. It also includes a marker sometimes called 'race' – which may be expressed as the potential to encounter discrimination or harassment based on a racialized description of that identity. This is not a trivial or inconsequential matter, although it may be contentious. It has had major consequences for all sectors of public service, from health to policing, and is of increasing importance as we move into the twenty-first century.

Ethnic monitoring can only be achieved and made valuable if health service workers, particularly those such as nurses and reception staff who have to collect the data, are comfortable with these concepts. They must understand the importance of language, religion and culture for health, and the importance of changing services to reflect the needs of a diverse population. Equally, they and their managers must be committed to using the information for the benefit of patients, and be prepared to take action when the data show inequality or inequity. Only then can they convince users of the need to provide the information they require to take these steps.

Clearly there are still questions to be asked and answered. The information revolution that is still affecting the NHS may yet provide answers. If, subject to the laws on data protection, ethnic category information can be collected in primary care, and the data can be stored in personal records that are passed to (and from) hospitals in referral letters and electronic files, this should reduce both work and friction caused by asking afresh every time the user encounters a service (Pringle and Rothera 1996). The same is true of other information. No-one seriously argues against recording date of birth, sex, or NHS identity numbers. In time, as the value of ethnic identity information is fed back into service planning and provision, it is to be hoped that the more we know, the better we can care. In the meanwhile, nurses need to be ready to explore the implications of diversity, and to offer their clients the opportunity to express their needs in terms of their ethnic identity for that monitoring.

PART II

Ethnicity and practice

5 Nursing, culture and competence

Lorraine Culley

Introduction

Several recent health policy directives emphasize the need for a healthcare practice which can address the health disadvantage which is experienced by some members of minority ethnic communities (Department of Health 1997, 1998d; Acheson 1998). Nursing is clearly identified as central to the delivery of these objectives. This chapter examines the debate about the role which culture plays in health inequalities and discusses how nursing has constructed the issue of multicultural healthcare. The chapter uses examples from recent research to illustrate the problems with a simplistic interpretation of the role of culture in health and healthcare. It provides some critical comment on the concept of transcultural nursing, while at the same time insisting on the importance of developing cultural competence as one component of improving services to minority ethnic communities.

The role of culture in explaining health inequalities

There has been a great deal of debate surrounding the possible role which cultural factors might play in understanding differences in health status between ethnic groups. For some, the suggestion that cultural differences may be implicated in explaining health inequalities is merely a diversion from the 'real' source of divisions in socio-economic differences and/or racism. Others however, while recognizing the dangers of explanations which ignore the socio-political context, argue that it is nevertheless important for appropriate healthcare interventions to be informed by an understanding of people's values, beliefs and customs. It is certainly the case that socio-economic inequalities are of major significance for health status (Acheson 1998). While this is widely acknowledged to be relevant for the population as a whole, the relationship between socio-economic status and health for minority ethnic communities has been given much less attention. It is often assumed in medical epidemiological research for example, that ethnicity in itself, will be the determining factor in explaining health inequalities (Sheldon and Parker 1992). However, more recently, the comprehensive community survey carried out by the Policy Studies Institute (Nazroo 1997a) has provided detailed evidence of health status which allows us to compare ethnic groups and to take into account differences of socio-economic status, age and gender and the effects these might have.

This study showed that the relatively deprived position of many ethnic minority groups compared with whites, contributes significantly to their poorer health and that controlling for standard of living gave a large improvement in the health of minority ethnic groups compared with whites. However, this does not mean that ethnic differences can be reduced to social class differences. As Smaje (1996) has argued, the ethnic patterning of health cannot be explained purely on the grounds of socio-economic disadvantage (see also Chapter 2, this volume). There is an interaction of material and cultural factors which must themselves be located in the wider context of a racist society.

Unfortunately, this interaction of cultural, structural (e.g. poverty) and political factors (e.g. institutional racism) has received relatively little attention in the literature. When the health of minority ethnic communities is addressed, what have been termed 'culturalist' explanations (Ahmad 1996a) are more commonly proposed. Culture is invoked as an explanation for health behaviour and health inequalities.

There are however, several problems associated with the way in which a simplistic concept of culture has been invoked as an explanation for health variations between ethnic groups. As several commentators have pointed out (Stubbs 1993; Ahmad 1993, 1996a; Culley 1997) culture is often conceived of as a fixed and unchanging property (or essence) of individuals or groups. This essentialist concept of culture is then seen to map onto ethnic groups, so that ethnic groups are defined as cultural groups – manifesting particular sets of cultural attributes or traits. In this view, culture and thereby ethnicity, is seen as something which is rigid and constraining and as something which mechanistically determines the behaviour of ethnic groups.

There are many who have criticized this notion of culture and its effects. One of the fiercest critics of the culturalist approach to health and healthcare is Waqar Ahmad (Ahmad 1996a) and it is worth outlining the main thrust of his argument in some detail. Ahmad draws on the critique of 'new racism' which is based on ideas of cultural difference. Cultural or 'new racism' (see Chapter 1) builds on a long historical tradition of the ideological justification for colonial domination in which the culture of the colonized was presumed to be inferior to the 'civilized' culture of the white middle classes and still today plays an important part in the strategy of control of black people's lives. Ahmad charts the way in which professional ideologies in health and social welfare construct and reinforce cultural differences as the source of health problems. Cultural understanding and cultural re-socialization (into the norms of the white society) are posited as the solution to health inequalities. Authors such as Qureshi (1989) and Rack (1990) have constructed notions of culturally cohesive communities with broadly negative stereotypes.

> The world of culture and medicine in relation to minority ethnic communities is largely the world of these lifeless, limp, cellophane-wrapped and neatly tagged cultures, rather than one of living and lived in cultures with all their vitality, complexity, complementarities and contradictions, cultures that are empowering, changing, challenging and flexible – cultures that are real. (Ahmad 1996a: 199)

Cultures, defined in rigid and static terms, come to be classified as either British or 'alien' and people are thus defined as more or less 'other' and more or less belonging. 'West Indians', for example, are stereotypically described as resentful of authority, having low educational standards and being involved in drugs and crime. Asian families are seen as close-knit and industrious but very different culturally. In recent years Muslims in particular have been characterized as alien and intolerant fanatics who pose a threat to the 'British way of life'.

Ahmad goes on to argue that the notion that behaviour is structured according to culturally based health beliefs in a direct and linear way is false. He also argues that there are significant 'cultural' differences between people who are typically defined as part of a cultural group. There is considerable evidence of diversity in the beliefs and behaviours within defined ethnic groups and there is considerable convergence between beliefs and customs across cultural groups and across countries.

As an example of this point Ahmad discusses the very different ways in which childbirth is experienced by three Pakistani Muslim women. The first woman is from a rich, middle class metropolitan background and her maternity care is highly medicalized and very similar to that received by women of similar social class in the UK. The second is a village woman who is cared for by a local traditional birth attendant and who observes the range of religious and cultural proscriptions associated with the 40-day recuperation period (chilla). This is further contrasted with the experience of a woman who provides hard physical labour on road construction. This women works until shortly before the birth and returns to work a few days later, not because she does not recognize the importance of the chilla, but because the economic situation of the family means that she must continue to contribute to the family income. All three are Muslim women in present-day Pakistan and are part of Pakistani culture on childbirth, yet because of the differences of social class, of rural/urban location and access to healthcare, their lives and experiences of birth are very different. Here Ahmad is illustrating the significance of structural issues such as socioeconomic status and spatial location interacting with 'culture' or tradition to produce different healthcare experiences.

We can see in this example how social class in particular will be significant in how a 'Muslim culture' will be constructed in different contexts. This shows how ethnicity cannot be treated as a fixed property of individuals, shaping behaviour in a deterministic way. 'We are all ethnic, yet our ethnicity does not define us. We all need our ethnic identity to be respected, yet we cannot be adequately understood solely in terms of our ethnicity' (Gerrish *et al.* 1996: 19). Ethnic identity is overlaid with gender, age, socio-economic and professional identities, each of which may be more or less significant in any specific context or at any specific point in time. Yet there is a tendency to define black people in particular solely by their supposed ethnicity. We rarely identify white people as a cultural group or sub-group. Majority ethnicity is under-theorized and under-researched. Indeed one consequence of a culturalist approach is that the alleged cultural attributes of minority ethnic groups are usually contrasted with an ethnic majority (the white population) which is itself seen as largely undifferentiated in cultural terms. As several commentators have pointed out, a moment's reflection shows that it is difficult to sustain the notion of a homogenous 'white' British culture. This false notion has, however, played a role in the relative invisibility of 'white' minority groups such as the Irish (Greenslade *et al.* 1997).

The culturalist approach then, tends to regard ethnic groups as homogenous, failing to recognize the significance of differences of class, gender, age and other statuses *within* broadly defined ethnic groups. This is exacerbated by research which seeks out an 'ethnic effect' while failing to take into consideration the influence of socio-economic or other statuses which we know to be very relevant to health. This is particularly evident in epidemiological research (Sheldon and Parker 1992; Sashidhran and Francis 1993; Ahmad 1996a). In such research there is a danger that differences *between* ethnic groups become overemphasized while differences *within* ethnic groups are ignored. At the same time *similarities* between the experiences of different ethnic groups (especially between minority ethnic and 'white' groups) often remain unexplored.

These issues are further illustrated in two pieces of research which examine different accounts of how people perceive and manage their illness. First, the work of Lambert and Sevak on perceptions of coronary heart disease (CHD) among groups of South Asian origin in London shows that perceptions of risk, CHD and ways of maintaining health were broadly similar among a number of Asian sub-groups. This work also suggests that a comparison with studies of UK residents of 'white' British origin would reveal that the major contrast is not between different ethnic groups but between biomedical and lay health cultures generally (Lambert and Sevak 1996). Second, a study of Asian and white stroke survivors carried out in Leicester showed that their experiences of stroke were similar. Both groups reported shortcomings in the information provided on recovery and the range of services available in the community and both groups had difficulties in identifying professionals responsible for their care (Perry *et al.* 1999). The point here is not that cultural differences in health beliefs and health behaviours do not exist, but that they cannot be assumed. The existence or otherwise of cultural differences and their correspondence to ethnic affiliation must be a matter of empirical investigation rather than seen as a self-evident fact (Lambert and Sevak 1996).

Even if significant differences of perception were shown to exist in a sample population, there would be a danger in generalizing from this to all members of an ethnic group and to all times and places, since an ethnic group does not have a unitary culture, and all cultures change over time. Culture is dynamic and contextual (Ahmad 1996a), not rigid and unchanging.

In defence of 'culture'

As we have seen, what has been described as the 'culturalist' perspective assumes a linear and mechanistic link between cultural beliefs and behaviour which cannot be theoretically or empirically sustained (Ahmad 1993) and it operates with a static and monolithic notion of culture which often results in crude stereotypes, categorizing cultural traits and applying them to particular ethnic groups. Being critical of such notions however, does not mean that we should discard all notions of culture as irrelevant to health. Kelleher (1996), for example, has forcefully argued in defence of culture and ethnicity. Kelleher acknowledges the potential danger of stereotyping but argues that this should be avoidable and that there are many benefits to an improved understanding of cultural influences on health behaviour. He accepts the criticisms of essentialist views of culture, but argues that how individuals respond to the threat of illness, the experience of illness and treatment regimens is affected by a host of factors, including the taken-for-granted ideas of their culture. People selectively draw on cultural elements to help them manage the situations they face: 'Ethnographic studies of the living, changing culture of particular ethnic groups will help us to understand their behaviour and to shape our own

accordingly' (Kelleher 1996: 85). Social research can identify
what people see as relevant in the day-to-day management of
their lives and contextualize these within the political and economic structures which shape their lives (p. 88). Unfortunately,
health research which meets these criteria is relatively scarce.

Those who reject the idea of defining ethnic groups in terms
of sets of fixed cultural attributes, stress the malleability of
ethnic identity, its changing nature and the fact that ethnicity
is situational. By this is meant that as the individual moves
through daily life, ethnicity can change according to the variations in the situations and the audiences encountered (Wallman
1986). Ethnic identities are themselves constantly evolving.
There are those who refer to the 'new ethnicities', which are
hybrids – the ever-changing products of complex processes of
social change (Hall 1992). In the postmodern view, ethnic identities are subject to change, redefinition and contestation. They
are not stable or permanent orderings of people, and individuals are not the bearers of culture, but the active creators of
culture. This 'social constructionist' approach to ethnicity and
cultural differentiation involves an appreciation that ethnic
identity is situationally variable and negotiable (see Chapter 1,
this volume).

However, to insist that ethnic identity may be changeable
does not mean that it always is or has to be. Ethnicity is not
always in a state of flux and may be more or less flexible in different times and places. One reason for this relates to the role
that social *categorization* plays in ethnicity and the importance
of relationships of power and domination (Jenkins 1997).
Ethnic boundaries are not just a matter of internal definition,
they are also constructed by outside agents and organizations.
Ethnic identification is not simply a matter of personal choice.
External forces such as immigration policies, census and other
ethnic categories, social policy legislation and so on are part of
this process. Personal and social identities are created in the
meeting of internal and external definitions. Power and authority relations are very important here, since some individuals
and groups are in a more powerful position than others to
impose a characterization (and name or category) on others in
a way which affects their social experience in significant ways.
An extreme form of this was in the South African system of

apartheid, but more subtle forms of social categorization and social exclusion exist in all societies.

Culture, structure and service provision

The chapter so far has argued that an essentialist view of ethnic identity can obscure some important issues in explanations of health differences. When we consider the delivery of health-care, equally damaging effects are evident. The culturalist approach can lead to a politics of 'victim-blaming' in which minority ethnic communities are seen as dangerous to their own health because they are seen to have cultural attributes which are not only different (or 'other') but pathological (Pearson 1986b). Some authors have shown how this can lead to minority groups themselves being perceived as problematic rather than the problem being located in ethnocentric health services (Douglas 1995). Ill health is seen emanating from primarily cultural attributes (such as dietary habits or restrictions on physical activity) rather than from structural factors such as poverty, social exclusion or racism. It has been argued that this kind of approach was apparent in the attempts to 'resocialize the culturally deviant' in campaigns such as the *Stop Rickets* and *Asian Mother and Baby* campaigns of the 1970s and the 1980s (Rocheron 1988) and to some extent in more recent debates about consanguinity and health problems in the Pakistani community (Ahmad 1994). Interestingly, cultural practices which could be said to be health promoting (e.g. vegetarian diets) and supportive and protective aspects of cultural identity are invariably ignored (Smaje 1995a).

Both cultural and structural factors are likely to be of significance in any understanding of health phenomena. This interaction is well illustrated in a qualitative study of iron deficiency anaemia in women of South Asian descent in north-west England which highlights the interplay of cultural and structural factors (Chapple 1998). Women of South Asian descent suffer relatively high levels of iron deficiency anaemia and this has been assumed to be primarily dietary in origin and thus resolvable by dietary adjustment. However, interviews with thirteen women of South Asian descent who were experiencing 'excessive' menstrual blood loss (menorrhagia) which significantly increases the incidence of anaemia, discovered a more complex set of factors involved. The research found that the women valued heavy menstrual periods, because this signifies the cleansing of the inner body and a return to normal body shape. It was also found that where dietary modifications were made to attempt to reduce the effects of blood loss they tended to exclude foods characterized as 'hot' such as meat and fish, which would actually add to the danger of iron deficiency. However, in addition to what might be regarded as 'cultural' issues, other factors clearly played a significant part in preventing appropriate treatment. In particular, the lack of female doctors and the lack of interpreters were major obstacles to seeking advice for menorrhagia and difficulties of communication of information about the condition led to some of the women not following medical advice and treatment. This study shows the significance of cultural values but it also highlights the impact of inadequate service provision – in this case the supply of female doctors and the provision of interpreters and advocates.

In some cases, the structural factors which surround health care provision may be the key feature in some forms of disadvantage experienced by minority ethnic communities in some contexts. A study of the provision of district nursing services by Gerrish (1999) illustrates the significance of structural barriers to service provision. Previous research has suggested that the relatively low up-take of district nursing services may relate to a reluctance of GPs to refer patients or a lack of demand on the part of patients, possibly because of lack of cultural sensitivity in service provision. This study highlighted very marked inequalities in district nursing provision between different GP practices. Single-handed, inner-city GP practices with a large minority ethnic practice population received a much smaller allocation of nursing staff than single group practices serving a smaller and predominantly white practice population. This was largely found to be an effect of institutional forces which determined the allocation of resources. In the absence of additional funding, the fund-holding GPs in large group practices were able to exert influence to prevent any redistribution of resource. The minority ethnic communities with a preponderance of (non-fund-holding) single handed practices were marginalized. As Gerrish points out, in these circumstances, even if district nurses were to develop more culturally sensitive practice and individual racism were eliminated, there are powerful institutional and structural forces at work which serve to perpetuate the disadvantage experienced by minority ethnic communities.

Research carried out among the Chinese community in Manchester (Chan 2000) provides a further illustration of the relevance of non-cultural factors. This study showed that although there were aspects of health beliefs which impacted on health behaviour, difficulties of poverty and social deprivation, the limited knowledge of the Chinese community on the part of health professionals and problems of communication in the absence of interpreters were found to be very significant issues affecting the quality of primary healthcare.

Ethnicity and nursing practice

One effect of an essentialist view of culture is that it tends to lead to a 'deficit' theory which attributes the social difficulties of minorities to the inadequacy of their cultural resources. One possible consequence of a culturalist approach for nursing is that it encourages the practice of negative stereotyping. Inappropriate and problematic concepts of culture and ethnicity may result in the development of crude stereotypes which categorize cultural traits and apply them to particular ethnic groups. Such a process leads to damaging encounters between healthcare personnel and minority ethnic users. Several studies have provided evidence of healthcare professionals portraying negative attitudes to clients from minority ethnic groups across a range of provision in primary/community services (Ahmad *et al.* 1991; Pharoah 1995), maternity services (Bowler 1993a; Hayes 1995), mental health services (Fernando 1991; Bhugra and Bahl 1999), health promotion (Douglas 1995) disability services (Ahmad 2000) and in social services provision (Ahmad and Atkin 1996). Although there is evidence of progress, some health professionals are failing to provide appropriate care to clients from minority ethnic groups (Thomas and Dines 1994; Rudat 1994; Gerrish *et al.* 1996). Two examples from nursing and midwifery research will serve as illustrations of how this can operate in practice to seriously disadvantage patients and clients.

Bowler (1993a) reports the findings of an ethnographic study which investigated the midwifery care of minority ethnic women of South Asian descent in a teaching hospital in southern England. The data were derived from interviews with 25 midwives and observations of interactions. The results showed that the midwives held a number of negative stereotypes of 'Asian' women. These included the view that Asian women were deviant in a number of ways. They were regarded as a homogenous group by the midwives based on their physical appearance (although the patients observed were in fact very heterogeneous in terms of cultural and religious background). They were typified generally as 'bad' patients. The women were described as unintelligent, as non-compliant, as abusers of the health service, having low pain thresholds, 'making a fuss about nothing' in labour, attention-seeking and lacking a normal maternal instinct.

Bowler's study reveals ways in which stereotypes affected the interaction between staff and women and how this interaction reinforced the negative views of women. There are several ways in which such stereotypes can disadvantage women. Bowler highlights the reluctance or inability of the midwives to communicate effectively with the women concerning fertility control after delivery because of assumptions that they would not be interested. She also suggests that women were not offered pain control in labour possibly because they were widely regarded as having easier deliveries than white women. These stereotypes persisted even in the face of evidence to the contrary. For example, one woman who had been taken down to the labour ward was being sought by the researcher. The midwife remarked 'Oh she'll be back in an hour, they're always quick'. This was despite the fact that the midwife was aware that the woman was having her first baby and being induced (both indicating the likelihood of a longer labour). In the event, the women had a slow and long labour.

The negative impact of stereotyping can also be seen in a study reported by Chiu *et al.* (1999). This study examined the participation of minority ethnic women in cervical screening programmes. Low up-take of screening has been attributed to health beliefs. However, research has tended to neglect other factors which may affect up-take, such as women's experience of and satisfaction with the screening service itself. This study of cervical smear takers and minority ethnic women patients, revealed a divergence in perceptions held by both groups regarding cervical screening, which contributed to negative experiences of the process. Focus group discussions with the smear takers revealed the existence of negative stereotyping of what were viewed as cultural mores and behaviours of Muslim women and men. South Asian women were seen as docile and lacking independence because of a male-dominated culture; they were seen as not having an understanding of preventative measures and reluctant to receive health education because of their culture. The smear takers thought that health education was a 'Western idea' rejected by the Asian community. 'Non-Westernized' women were seen as a problem with 'their' language and culture understood as barriers to effective medical practice: 'In general, stereotypes seemed to operate as a convenient justification for shifting the responsibility to minority ethnic women for lack of communication and opportunistic health education during smear taking' (Chiu *et al.* 1999: 11).

The research included mini-focus group discussions with 27 minority ethnic women clients, conducted by a specifically trained bilingual moderator. These revealed that the knowledge of many of the women about the purpose and procedure of the cervical smear test remained patchy. Despite the popular perception that the women were not interested in preventive healthcare, the participants were very keen to obtain information and explanations. All but one of the women had had smears taken (mostly opportunistically in the context of post-natal examination), but few had been given any explanation of the exact nature of the procedure or its purpose. Their experiences of having the test were overwhelmingly negative. For example, one woman, although accompanied by her English-speaking daughter reported that she was simply instructed to 'Get your pants down and get on the couch' (p. 16). Another woman reported 'I took my clothes off but I was very embarrassed and shaking and I had no idea what was this all about and why. So the nurse asked me to lie down. I put my legs together and didn't want to take the test. The nurse held my legs apart and took the test' (p. 16). Only one of the women had received any information about the procedure during their smear test. Some said they would like to know but could not ask because of language difficulties. In the absence of interpreters many women used their husbands as interpreters and this was perceived by the smear takers as further evidence of subordination, which in turn was seen as a barrier to up-take.

The study concluded that 'Smear takers in this study viewed minority culture as static, unified wholes and largely ignored the variations that exist between individuals. This failure to accept difference underpinned their negative views of minority ethnic women. Dysfunctional communication between smear takers and minority ethnic women appears to have been caused by stereotyping and the lack of knowledge and skills in intercultural encounters on the part of the smear takers. This is turn may lead to the dignity and confidentiality of women being compromised and engender feelings of helplessness and negativity' (Chiu *et al.* 1999: 16).

'Transcultural' nursing

As we have seen, one of the major errors of the culturalist approach is the conflation of ethnicity and culture. That is, ethnic groups are defined as cultural groups, which can be defined by stable sets of core cultural attributes – particular norms, values, beliefs and lifestyles. Thus one hears of an Asian culture, or Indian culture, or African-Caribbean culture and so on. However, as we have seen, such a view has been seriously challenged. Many sociologists today reject the notion of ethnicity as culture and ethnic groups as cultural groups. Culture and identity are part of the building blocks of ethnicity, as a social construction. But ethnicity is not an 'immutable bundle of cultural traits which it is sufficient to enumerate in order to identify a person as an "X" or a "Y"' (Jenkins 1997: 52).

This limited and unhelpful notion of cultural groups is especially manifest in the American approach to transcultural nursing pioneered by Leininger (1978) and is one of the major drawbacks to the 'factfile' approach to 'cultural sensitivity'. The American transcultural nursing movement has been heavily criticized for its view of culture as a unified whole with a direct causal link to behaviour. It has also been criticized as lacking an examination of the wider political and economic context which impacts upon health care and failing to adequately incorporate the experiences of racism into its model of cultural sensitivity (Bruni 1988; Alleyne *et al.* 1994; Mulholland 1995; Culley 1996). A similar problem arises with the use of ethnic 'factfiles' in the UK context. In such Lonely Planet Guides to ethnic minority health (Gerrish *et al.* 1996), groups are categorized according to religious or cultural beliefs and practices – dietary norms, language, naming systems, personal hygiene norms, rituals surrounding birth and death and so on (Qureshi 1989; Karmi 1992; Bal and Bal 1995). There has been very little evaluation of the effectiveness of these resources in nursing practice.

One study which has commented extensively on the use of factfiles is Gunaratnam's research on palliative care (Gunaratnam 1997; Gunaratnam *et al.* 1998). Gunaratnam argues that factfiles portray a one-dimensional snapshot of cultural practices, which are frozen in time and context and she argues that packaging cultural practices in this way can lead to practitioners actually bypassing the need to engage with the subjective experience and personal choice of users. She shows how a preoccupation with cultural identity can serve to limit professional intervention as multicultural practice becomes highly task-orientated. At the same time, because religious and other needs are portrayed as rigid and non-negotiable (e.g. 'Muslims eat these foods'), personal choice can be denied for patients. Dilemmas can be created for staff when individuals make demands and choices which contradict the alleged cultural traits and prescriptions. Gunaratnam also observed that professional anxieties about 'getting it wrong' were heightened and practice was therefore channelled into 'safe' but often unimaginative areas.

The factfile approach fails to recognize that nursing in a diverse society can be stressful and challenging as well as highly rewarding. Not least because there are many wider structural issues which are outside the immediate context of the nursing encounter, which can have a major impact on the relationship of nurse and patient/user. Inappropriate ethnic monitoring processes, inadequate or non-existent facilities for translation and interpreting, heavy workloads which make taking extra time to discuss care difficult, can all impact on the relationship of nurse and patient. If one adds to this the background of a society which manifests many forms of racisms both personal and institutional, it is not surprising that both professional and patient anxieties can be raised. Gunaratnam's study also highlighted that staff had many fears about confronting their own and other people's racisms and that factfiles are silent on how to deal with such issues.

Becoming competent – tensions and dilemmas

Competent nursing practice must include being able to negotiate care in an encounter where at least some of the beliefs, values, attitudes and experiences of nurse and patient differ. The examples outlined earlier in the chapter show the consequences for patients when practitioners are not able to deliver care in a competent and culturally safe manner. But it must be recognized that because ethnic groups are not unifed cultural wholes, because culture is complex and changing, because ethnic identity is to some degree situational and dynamic and because we live in a racist society, the task of providing good care is itself complex and fraught with difficulty. The nurse faces a tension between the need to recognize and respond to cultural difference and the necessity of doing this without recourse to stereotyping. This will require a number of skills, which nurses must work towards developing if they are to manage cross-cultural encounters efficiently.

Gerrish *et al.* (1996) have outlined the ways in which nurses can work towards ensuring an effective and sensitive mode of interpersonal communication. Drawing on the work of Kim (1992) the authors suggest that there may be generic communicative skills which can be learned and which prepare individuals to be optimally flexible and adept at meeting the challenge of intercultural interactions, regardless of the specific cultures involved in the exchange. This they refer to as 'intercultural communicative competence'. Adaptability (cognitive, affective and behavioural) is at the heart of this competence: 'It involves the acquisition of a cognitive style and an attitudinal stance towards "the stranger" which prevents the practitioners from artificially and hastily reducing the ambiguity present in the encounter. It enables the practitioner to work with that ambiguity through an open and empathetic negotiation of the client's identity and needs. This competence must surely exist as a necessary range of abilities characteristic of any practitioner who claims to offer holistic care' (p. 29). Such generic skills would go a long way to providing effective communication with clients.

In some contexts, it might also be appropriate for nurses to acquire more specific knowledge about what possible aspects of a client's ethnic identity and cultural background might have a bearing on healthcare. This may present the nurse with a dilemma. Practitioners must avoid stereotypes, but must have sufficient prior knowledge to know what *might* be relevant to the caring encounter. The danger of stereotyping is real, yet professionals require the knowledge base to anticipate what particular beliefs, religious or other cultural prescriptions etc. *may* have relevance so that appropriate forms of care can be negotiated. Lack of such knowledge can lead not only to personal distress and offence but may have serious consequences for treatment. It is helpful therefore, to be aware of possible issues to explore with clients, without assuming that they are inevitably of significance. As Gunaratam argues (this volume) ambiguity should be recognized as a fundamental characteristic of multicultural work – there are no certainties of practice which are going to be relevant at all times. Nursing must allow flexibility of response and not seek permanent 'solutions'. Abandoning the notion of fixed homogenous cultures, means that nurses must be prepared to 'get it wrong' as well as to try to 'get it right'.

Rejecting what we have called essentialist views of culture does not mean rejecting the idea that aspects of culture can influence health and healthcare. However, nurses need to use communication skills to *ascertain* rather than *assume* what preferences and practices are of significance to patients. They must recognize the importance of not just ethnic differences, but the significance of other identities relating to class, sexuality and generation for example. To refer to a patient as 'Asian', tells us very little that could be of any use to the nurse in providing appropriate healthcare, any more than referring to a patient as 'white' would. Nurses need to seek information which might be relevant to healthcare practice – what religious needs patients might have, what foods they prefer to eat, how they prefer to wash and what the patient's own narrative of their illness is. Listening to the patient's story, exploring with them the ways in which aspects of their ethnic identity might be significant in their lives and in their response to illness and working to build partnerships with patients are more important than learning lists of alleged cultural norms. An essential part of good nursing care is the ability to recognize that many people feel anxious and stressed when they are in a medical environment. Nurses need to reflect on the additional stress which might be felt by people who have little English or who find British hospitals bewildering or who feel rejected because of their ethnic origin (Henley 1991).

Reflection is a tool which most nurses are taught to use. A useful first step for nurses is to reflect upon a hypothetical situation in which they find themselves to be ill in another country, one where perhaps they have only a little knowledge of the healthcare system and little facility with the dominant language. What would you most like the staff caring for you to know about you? Reflecting on this might suggest to the nurse a number of aspects of care which would be relevant. Henley (1991) provides a useful set of guidelines which cover some of the practical aspects of caring for minority ethnic patients. Areas to explore with clients include questions about food (e.g. religious and personal preferences, fasting); physical care (e.g. how patients like to keep clean, hair care, significance of jewellery); physical exposure (e.g. ensuring physical modesty, explaining routine procedures, ensuring hospital gowns cover areas of the body some women find it offensive to bare in public); spiritual care (e.g. asking if and how religion is important to patients); caring for dying patients and their families (e.g. having access to information about likely preferences related to care around time of death); names and records (e.g. getting a patients full name, finding out how they would like to be addressed, achieving correct pronunciation). To avoid stereotyping, Henley offers the following advice to nurses: 'Your guiding principle should be *never assume, always ask*. Never assume from a patient's name or appearance or religion what their needs are. Ask sensitive questions and treat any patient's wishes and feeling in the way you would like your own to be treated' (Henley 1991: 6).

Some of the most challenging encounters for nurses will occur where there is a language difference between caregiver and receiver. Nurses require training in making the best use of professional interpreters where these are available. However, facilities for effective interpretation are woefully inadequate in the NHS. It is crucial that while arguing for more professional resources to be provided, nurses also need to be trained to facilitate communication across a language barrier in the absence of interpreters (see Chapter 6, this volume).

Those who have been rightly critical of a culturalist approach have stressed the importance of an awareness of 'race' and racialization. It is essential that the need to understand and listen to patients includes the need to understand racism and its effects. Recognizing and challenging racism is often difficult and uncomfortable. There are additional dilemmas for staff when they are faced with racist behaviour from patients and clients in their care. The NHS has an obligation to assist nurses to discuss these issues in a sensitive manner, to provide space for nurses to confront their own exclusionary values and practices and to provide training in how to respond appropriately to racisms on the part of patients and colleagues.

Conclusion

The chapter has argued that the way in which cultural difference has often been invoked in health and nursing research and practice is problematic and can lead to potentially damaging effects for minority ethnic patients and clients. It has also argued that there is an equal danger in failing to recognize the potential impact of cultural differences on the delivery of healthcare. Developing skills in the delivery of healthcare in a culturally diverse and dynamic society may be challenging and difficult but is essential for all healthcare workers. The chapter has also attempted to show that while it is appropriate to take account of the potential impact of culture on health and to stress the need for cultural competence in nursing, such factors must be seen as one set of influences among many. Improving individual nursing practice is only one element in a wider set of changes required to improve the healthcare experiences of minority ethnic groups. In addition to improving cultural competence in their own practice, nurses can play a wider role in the transformation of health provision towards a more participative model, which takes the views of users seriously and seeks to develop services through working with communities. With the current emphasis on primary care and the explicit commitment to reducing inequalities in health, community health nurses in particular are in a good position to work with others towards public health models and community development approaches which many commentators see as the way forward (Acheson 1998). An awareness of the historical positioning of minority ethnic communities in British society, the structural and organizational barriers to equitable healthcare and ways of challenging these must be a central part of the educational preparation of nurses for the twenty-first century.

It has not been possible in to discuss at any length the implications of this analysis for nurse education. Research evidence has shown that currently nurse education is in many cases failing to prepare practitioners to provide culturally competent care, despite the fact that both the UKCC and the ENB have requirements which include statements about the preparation for practice in a multicultural society (Le Var 1998). There is no shortage of useful ideas about how pre- and post-registration nurse education (in both educational and practice settings) needs to be fundamentally reviewed to encourage and enable the development of a nursing workforce which can work more effectively within an ethnically diverse society (Culley 1996, 1997; Le Var 1998; Gerrish *et al.* 1996; Gerrish 1997; Baxter 1998; Lister 1999). Education for cultural diversity should not be seen as a simple or easily achievable process. To be effective it must be able to challenge and overcome resistances, both personal and institutional: 'Our biases, prejudices, and stereotypes run deep and die hard!' (Sue 1994).

6 Communication, interpretation and translation

Hannah Bradby

Introduction

This chapter considers communication in health settings, with particular reference to cases where the health service provider speaks a different language from the patient. The context is set by reviewing the global dominance of the English language and the relative power of health professionals and patients who might be involved in a multilingual encounter. Barriers to communication include speaking different languages, different varieties of language and holding various expectations of an encounter, all of which may be related to mismatches between patient and health practitioner in terms of ethnicity, age, gender, class, nationality or professional background.

Communication barriers in healthcare settings need to be tackled on two levels: first, at the level of national policy, including consideration of nurse and midwifery education and accreditation; and second, at the level of routine individual interactions between health practitioners and patients. This chapter focuses on the second of these levels and the ways that interpretation, in its broadest sense, is needed to overcome barriers. Interpretation between health professionals and patients might involve acting in an advocacy role, particularly where communication is blocked by racism or other discrimination. Brief consideration is given to how advocacy combines with nursing and when it is more appropriately taken on by a non-nurse.

Finally, strategies available for interpretation between languages in healthcare settings are reviewed. Lack of resources for interpretation services undoubtedly compromises the quality of healthcare provision, but linguistic interpretation is not the only aspect of competent cross-cultural communication. Equally crucial is that health professionals be aware of the peculiarities of their own professional culture and the necessity of interpreting for patients who do not share their professional assumptions, nor other aspects of background, such as religion, family structure and education.

Power – English as a dominant language

English is a prestigious language, in that it is the second most widely spoken language in the world and has become the dominant language in international relations and science (Grillo 1989; Venuti 1995), including medicine and nursing. The history of the rise of English is related to Britain's history of colonial (Alladina 1993) and mercantile expansionism (Wardhaugh 1987; Grillo 1989) and has been maintained into the twenty-first century through the widespread use of English in computing. The twentieth century prosperity of Britain's former colonies, such as the USA, Canada, Australia and New Zealand, attracts migrants from less affluent countries in search of educational and occupational opportunities. At the time when industrialized countries such as Britain were receiving the peak number of labour migrants, many had also instituted forms of state-provided welfare programmes such as the National Health Service (NHS), available to migrants, but generally without provision for multilingual communities.

Problems facing migrants to English-speaking countries were not only the lack of provision for interpretation in health services, but also the low esteem in which minority languages were held. The languages of racialized minorities are often viewed as being less cultivated than English to the point that British educational policy has regarded minority languages spoken at home as an impediment to the learning of English (Linguistic Minorities Project 1985; Rampton 1995). This view ignores the ancient and considerable literature associated with the Sanskrit traditions of Hindi and the Persian traditions of Urdu, sister languages to many of those spoken by British Asians, such as Gujarati, Punjabi and Bengali.

Communication in health care settings

Communication is a complex process, not reducible to its linguistic component alone. Successful interpersonal communication necessitates the interpretation of speech, tone and register of language, facial expressions, body language, gestures and assumptions shared between the communicants about the context and purpose of the exchange (Quill 1989; Chapman 1995; Baylav 1996). As one nurse puts it, 'there's a whole lot more to communication than words' (Hatton and Webb 1993).

While the practice of nursing in general requires communication, it is particularly crucial to the process of diagnosis (Ebden *et al.* 1988). A nurse may be called upon to aid a diagnosis through her linguistic as well as nursing skills. Nurses acting as interpreters are not uncommon in countries where they are more likely than doctors to speak the less prestigious languages (such as Spanish in the USA and Xhosa in South Africa), generally without reward for or recognition of the linguistic and clinical skills necessary to fulfil this task adequately (Drennan 1996). Outside the hospital, nurses are more likely to be in charge of diagnosing, referring and treating patients, and the limited literature that deals specifically with language and nursing mostly concentrates on the community setting (Wilson 1989; Hatton and Webb 1993; Wessel 1998).

The medical dominance (Freidson 1970) that structures discourse in clinical settings between doctors and nurses also has implications for communication between nurses and patients. The degree to which nurses collude with medical dominance and adopt the medical discourse is an issue at the heart of the ongoing development of the relationship between nursing and midwifery and medicine. Some commentators view a central role of nurse professionals as that of avoiding collusion with medical discourse, by adopting the role of advocate.

Patients from minority groups that have been subject to racialization (Bradby 1995), face a racist discourse, in addition to the medical discourse, which further constrains the possibilities for communication. Racism in its institutional and individual forms pervades many dimensions of the NHS (Ahmad 1992), including nurse–patient communication. Even

if nursing and midwifery as professions could utterly rid themselves of racism, in isolation from change in wider society, the
experience of racist exclusion and marginalization elsewhere
means that racialized patients are likely to interpret routine
misunderstandings or mistakes as confirmation of deliberate
exclusion (Gerrish *et al.* 1996). In circumstances such as a group
of patients facing economic deprivation, racism and not speaking English, a strong case for non-nurse advocates has been
made to improve particular health outcomes, such as those
around birth.

Effective communication with patients is a worthy goal in
and of itself. Evidence shows that not only is effective communication associated with compliance (Auerback 1995) and
patient satisfaction (Baker *et al.* 1998), but also with some improved health outcomes (Meryn 1998). Conversely, poor
service provider communication constitutes a significant barrier
to the receipt of good quality health care (Torres 1998), and is
associated with non-compliance with preventative services, even
after adjusting for socio-economic factors and contact with the
health services (Woloshin *et al.* 1997). An inability to speak
English in the USA, Britain and Australia is associated with a
range of indicators of the inappropriate use of various hospital
services (Wright 1994; Lee *et al.* 1998; Stolk *et al.* 1998) and
with children's poor health status (Stuart *et al.* 1996; Woloshin
et al. 1997). Ineffective communication is likely to lead to
worsening health outcomes, particularly with complex and/or
chronic health problems (Hornberger *et al.* 1997) and with
mental health problems, where the lack of a common language
can lead to misdiagnosis, ineffective, harmful treatment and
longer admissions (Stolk *et al.* 1998).

Good quality of nursing care necessitates that good communication, combined with cultural competency, be extended
towards all patients, routinely, by all members of the profession.
The nursing profession is not judged by the best practice of their
most competent members, but by the routine performance of
all members (Gerrish *et al.* 1996) and this observation can be
generalized to suggest that until society at large is no longer
racist then any profession, including nursing, must demonstrate
what Gerrish *et al.* call 'appropriate cultural knowledge and

an empathetic attitude towards minority ethnic clients' (p. 41) in order to counterbalance an expectation of hostility and marginalization.

Barriers to communication

The distress and pain which brings a patient to the health services can render communication even more difficult. The patient's ability to communicate in a non-native language and to overcome ignorant or prejudiced assumptions about his/her cultural or religious background may be severely reduced by the nature of their illness or injury (Stolk *et al.* 1998). This may be particularly true when communication is taking place in a stressful situation (Totten *et al.* 1996) dealing with sensitive issues, as is often the case in psychiatric and emergency services (Musser-Granski and Carrillo 1997; Lee *et al.* 1998). The problem of communicating with distressed people is not, of course, peculiar to patients who do not speak fluent English and the goal of effective communication ought to be a routine part of a health professional's work, regardless of the languages involved (Phelan and Parkman 1995).

In addition to spoken language, use can be made of written materials in appropriate languages to supplement and confirm aspects of clinical communication. Written communication is obviously less flexible than the spoken word, depending as it does on literacy. Pre-prepared leaflets on particular procedures or conditions exist, but, assuming they are appropriately translated from English originals (Naish *et al.* 1994), their usefulness depends on patients' literacy. In Britain rates of illiteracy are higher among some recently migrated populations, and an inability to read or write English does not necessarily imply literacy in the mother-tongue. For instance a survey found that among the Bangladeshi population of Leeds, 49 per cent were illiterate in English, and 35 per cent were also illiterate in Bengali (Tuffnell *et al.* 1994). In this case the provision of information sheets in Bengali would not be a total solution to communicating, for example, breast screening information (Hobbs *et al.* 1989). However, where literacy is confirmed, written materials can be useful because they can be removed and considered at length, after a consultation.

In day-to-day nursing work, written communication can only be of limited use and cannot compensate for an inability to speak with patients. Broader issues of communication between healthcare providers and patients, such as the use of patient-held records are raised by considering the needs of populations with a significant minority who cannot read or write English, or any other language. For the purpose of the current discussion which concentrates on spoken language, the following elements of communication will be considered: language, variety, dialect or idiom, and cultural and social expectations.

Language

Studies in Britain and other English-speaking countries have shown that a considerable proportion of clinical encounters occur between people who share no common language (Tuffnell *et al.* 1994; Wright 1994; Hornberger *et al.* 1996; Stuart *et al.* 1996; Hornberger *et al.* 1997; Woloshin *et al.* 1997; Lee *et al.* 1998; Stolk *et al.* 1998). Patients are meeting healthcare providers and relying on mime, gestures, minimal language and a variety of unsuitable interpreters including children. Clearly this is not satisfactory in that patients are not receiving adequate care, in that confidentiality is compromised, misdiagnosis risked and patients subject to undue embarrassment and stress. However, these problems are not necessarily due to the non-existence of trained interpreters. Where there is provision of trained interpreters in appropriate languages, the service may only exist during office hours (Jones and Gill 1998) and/or professionals are discouraged from using them for budgetary reasons (Stolk *et al.* 1998).

But even if expert medical interpreters were universally available and availed of, communication problems would not necessarily be eradicated, due to the aspects of communication that involve interpretation within rather than between languages.

Language variety

Where a nurse and a patient are both English-speaking it is assumed that there are no impediments to communication (Cave *et al*. 1995). However, the meaning of words also depends on social, cultural and historical traditions (Schulte 1996) such that interpretation of the same words can vary. This variation may coincide with religious, ethnic or other cultural divisions within a single language group as with the various groups who lay claim to the Irish language (Chriost and Aitchison 1998). Different religious and ethnic groups may have an accent, or system of notation for a single language that distinguishes them from one another, for example spoken Hindi and Urdu are mutually comprehensible but use quite different systems for writing (Wardhaugh 1986). The variation in accent and vocabulary between Urdu and Hindi may be exaggerated or minimized depending on the social and political context of the speech.

In addition to language varieties that coincide with ethnic and religious divisions, age, sex, gender, education and social class may also be reflected in the type, tone or style of language that is employed (Lucas and Ware 1977; Porter 1991). For instance the variety of English that a young student nurse uses with a senior colleague probably differs systematically from her style of speech when talking to other students. Speech varies with the context of the speech (e.g. lecture theatre against pub) and the characteristics of the speaker and how these are shared with other communicants.

'Standard English' articulated with 'received pronunciation' is seen as the 'correct' variety of the language. Health professionals, by virtue of extended exposure to education, are more likely than many of their patients to use this variety, at least in clinical settings. However, this should not imply that there exists a neutral variety of language which is free of accent or dialect. Everyone speaks with an accent or dialect, but some of these varieties are more widespread or more prestigious than others (American Speech-language Hearing Association Joint Subcommittee of the Executive Board on English Language Proficiency 1998).

Different professions have their own varieties of English, defined by vocabulary and idiom, including health professionals whose language should communicate with one another and with patients (Porter 1991). However, there are times when communication between professionals may be incomprehensible to the lay person in both spoken and written forms (Ravaioli 1997).

The vocabulary employed by health professionals may make an obvious barrier to patient comprehension. For instance, in discussing 'family planning' with young people, an adult professional was told that every term that he used for contraceptive practices and body parts differed from the terms with which the young people were familiar (Lucas and Ware 1977). However, employing colloquial terms does not guarantee comprehension, as illustrated by the case of Japanese women in London who reported that words such as 'poo', 'pee' and 'tummy bug' hindered communication in primary care consultations (Arai and Farrow 1995), as they were more familiar with formal terms such as 'faeces', 'urine' and 'infection'. Other terms were not colloquial, but nonetheless caused confusion. For instance, the question 'how are baby's motions?' elicited the response 'he can walk' (Arai and Farrow 1995).

Even where vocabulary and pronunciation are shared between clinician and patient, the meaning and implication of particular words may vary hugely and is only comprehensible in the cultural and social context of the speaker. An example of this centres on the meaning of the symptom 'nerves' to a patient for whom it legitimizes her position in her social world as a respectable, burdened, yet stoical householder in contrast to its meaning to a clinician (Davis 1984). At this point examples of difference in variety of language between nurse and patient become difficult to distinguish from examples of differing expectations.

Expectations

Health professionals and patients hold expectations of the process of an encounter and its outcome. These expectations have changed in recent history, whereby previous levels of respect and trust in medicine have been undermined. More recently, rising education levels and the consumer movement have led to more assertive and questioning patients (Gabe *et al.* 1994; Thomasma 1994). Trusting respect for clinicians may be more evident among patients who have migrated from areas where biomedical health care has been recently introduced and/or where healers and learned people are highly respected. This respect may be accompanied by an expectation of certainty from a health professional. For instance, Japanese women in London described great respect for their general practitioner and in return expected definite guidance from a consultation: disappointment ensued if this was not forthcoming (Arai and Farrow 1995). 'Exalted status' is said to be enjoyed by clinicians in the eyes of patients migrated from Vietnam and China. Such high status may enhance patient compliance, but can also present difficulties, for instance, when patients prefer to remain silent in the face of incomprehension of, or disagreement with a health professional to avoid showing disrespect (Vu 1996). Similarly some cultures, including those of India, Pakistan, Bangladesh, Sri Lanka and Latin America, consider a negative response to be disrespectful in some circumstances, particularly if directed towards a learned stranger, which could mean a reluctance to say 'no' to a health professional's routine question.

What constitutes a legitimate health concern varies both within and between language groups and can form a barrier to communication. Cultural variation exists in the ways that different peoples consider mental distress to be the legitimate concern of medical professionals. To Pathan women living in England, (un)happiness was in the hands of Allah and it was felt inappropriate to bring symptoms of misery to a health service provider, since unfortunate circumstances could not be altered through the NHS (Currer 1986). When help is sought for psychological distress, the means by which this distress is expressed varies by culture, with different 'languages of emotion' having developed in different cultures (Leff 1988; Fenton and Sadiq-Sangster 1996). When the language of emotion is not shared between patient and health service provider, communication and provision of care may be jeopardized. Among Punjabis in Glasgow psychological distress may be presented to health service providers as bodily rather than as psychological symptoms, which could lead to under-diagnosis of mental health problems (Williams *et al.* 1997).

Disparities of expectation and interpretation between patient and professional are apparent with demanding, difficult or deviant patients (and can be read as part of their pathology (Totten *et al.* 1996)), but they may also occur with those people who are 'appropriate' service users. A study of expressions commonly used by healthcare staff in the US suggested that no assumption of a common interpretation of a phrase such as 'going home from hospital soon' or 'it'll only hurt a little' can be made (Anonymous 1981). From this survey almost 90 per cent of doctors were found to interpret 'going home from hospital soon' to mean either 2–4 days or 'an indeterminate time'. This can be contrasted with almost 20 per cent of patients who considered the phrase to mean 'tomorrow'. Interpretations of 'it'll only hurt a little' ranged from 'a quick pinch' to 'it'll probably hurt a lot', the latter being the response of 20 per cent of patients but only 2 per cent of doctors.

Barriers to communication come in many forms. Perhaps the most obvious is where there is little or no common language between interlocutors. However, even when two speakers share a vocabulary and an accent, and come from the same cultural and ethnic background, if one is a health professional and other a patient, there is potential for not sharing the interpretation of the meaning of an exchange.

Overcoming communication problems

Communication between nurses and patients takes place in a social context, which is crucial for the understanding that both parties carry from an encounter. Aspects of this context are iniquitous with regard to minority ethnic group and/or non-English-speaking patients and should be challenged at the level of professional and national policy. Simultaneously there are aspects of the ways that language and concepts are interpreted between individual patient and health professional to which attention should be paid by individuals and professional bodies alike.

Anti-racism and multiculturalism

Exclusion and marginalization based on religion, culture and language may be experienced by patients from their health service providers. Communication may also be compromised by health professionals being 'culturally incompetent', that is unaware of the linguistic and other needs of other ethnic groups. Amelioration of health service delivery to minority ethnic patients should not be simply dependent on recruiting nurses from the appropriate minority ethnic and language groups for two reasons. First, nurses should be consulted on whether or not they wish to specialize in the health care needs of a particular ethnic group of patients, and if they bring linguistic or other skills to the job, these should be rewarded. At the same time, patients should receive good quality care regardless of their own or their carer's ethnic background and therefore all nurses should be taught using an anti-racist approach that engenders cultural competency.

Initiatives to rid nursing and midwifery of exclusionary and marginalizing practice have taken the form of guidelines issued by professional bodies to nurses (Henley 1991) and health managers (Gerrish *et al.* 1996; Mitchell *et al.* 1998) and efforts to develop the teaching and assessment of multiethnic nursing (McGee 1992; Gerrish *et al.* 1996). In the case of patient groups whose health outcomes are remarkably poor and who are subject to deprivation and discrimination, special initiatives have been formulated at a national level (McCabe and Rocheron 1985; Bahl 1987; Mason 1990). Such inequity must be tackled at the levels of national and professional policy as well as at the level of the individual practitioner.

Translation and interpretation

Individual health professionals are accountable for their own practice (Henley 1991), including communication. Effective communication, whether or not it is across a language barrier, requires interpretation, in the broadest sense of the word. Nurses need to communicate with all patients so that the meaning of words, whether or not they are translated into

another language, is reflected upon in the course of the conversation. In order to understand a patient's interpretation of an
exchange the professional must consider both the words being
used, but also the historical and cultural context of those words
(Schulte 1996). The form that a conversation between a professional and a patient needs to take (particularly if a third
party translator is also involved), is that of a dance (Hatton and
Webb 1993) whereby meaning and interpretation are constantly
renegotiated and refined. This model of interpretation within a
single language suggests that the nurse should act as a cultural
bridge, mediating between the cultural system of the patient and
the cultural system of the health service.

Nurses are ideally placed in the division of health care labour
to act as such 'natural mediators' because of their location and
position within the health care team (Mallik 1997a). This medi-
ation, or bridging work, is referred to as 'advocacy' and a debate
as to the suitability and practicality of nurses taking on advocacy
is ongoing in Britain and the US (Mallik 1997a, 1997b; Anderson 1998; Manton 1998). The advocacy debate does not refer
explicitly to the special needs of patients who do not speak
English but the advocacy role requires attention to communication and language. For instance, it has been suggested that
the use of jargon combined with a collusion with doctors' orders
compromises the nurse's advocacy role (Martin 1998) to the
detriment of the patient's interests. Advocacy is regarded as particularly important when there are cultural or generational differences between the staff and patients and research into the way
that nurses' language is understood by patients is recommended
(Ward-Collins 1998).

Another, related debate considers the role of non-nurse advocates for particular groups of patients whose needs were not
being adequately met in particular areas of health care. The
Asian Mother and Baby campaign used the term 'link-worker'
to describe non-clinicians from the same ethnic group as patients
(in this case of South Asian origin), employed as interpreters,
but also to represent the patient's best interests and negotiate
with clinicians on her behalf (Bahl 1987). It seems clear that
communication is improved by link-worker schemes (McCabe
and Rocheron 1985; Mason 1990), but whether this translates
into better uptake of ante-natal services (Mason 1990) or

improved obstetric outcomes, such as lower Caesarean section rates (Parsons and Day 1992) is not clear.

Effective interpretation is often only possible if religious and/or cultural reasons for a patient's reaction to particular questions or treatments be described to the health care provider, to supplement the translation of the patient's own speech (Wilson 1989; Haffner 1992; Hatton and Webb 1993). For example, a Spanish-speaking patient whose words were translated said that her abdominal pain subsided when she 'passed pens'. The additional knowledge that this is a colloquial term for 'passing wind' made more sense of her condition (Wilson 1989). Equally, supplementing the patient's understanding of a health professional's advice with the background reasons for a particular medical practice may be necessary. An example is the delicacy of interpreting the concept of 'vasectomy' in such a way as to avoid any implication of 'castration', which can be difficult in cultures which equate a man's fertility with his virility (Lucas and Ware 1977).

Communication may involve more than just verbal interpretation, as understanding the social context may explain what a patient cannot say. Women from cultures that have strict codes of modesty may be unwilling to describe intimate bodily problems in front of a male relative (Diaz-Duque 1982; Vu 1996). A woman presented three times at a clinic, always accompanied by her son as interpreter, and described vague, changing complaints which did not make sense to the physician. Only on the fourth visit, which her son could not attend, was a female interpreter called, and the woman able to describe what turned out to be a fistula in her rectum (Haffner 1992).

The need for a translator to offer cultural, as well as linguistic, interpretation of professionals' speech is particularly clear for those working in mental health (Dodd 1983; McIvor 1994; Musser-Granski and Carrillo 1997; Stolk *et al.* 1998) because conceptions of mental health and expressions of mental distress vary with culture and language (Leff 1988; Fenton and Sadiq-Sangster 1996), and some medical professionals encourage interpreters to lead the line of questioning in therapeutic interviews (Musser-Granski and Carrillo 1997).

The view of interpreters as professionals who are actively working with health care providers and patients (Baylav 1996;

Musser-Granski and Carrillo 1997) is not the only one. The alternative model recommends that the interpreter remains 'invisible' (Phelan and Parkman 1995; Venuti 1995; Baylav 1996) acting as a 'voice box' (Hatton and Webb 1993) for the clinician. The interpreter is 'used by' the professional (Baylav 1996), who should 'keep control of the consultation' (Phelan and Parkman 1995; Barsky 1996). The fear that interpreters may step beyond their neutral role and distort communication with a patient is not unusual (Ebden *et al.* 1988; Brafman 1995).

There may be times when a neutral, invisible form of interpretation is appropriate, for instance, when there are legal implications to what the nurse is saying as in cases of suspected abuse. However it is not a means of working that is recommended or preferred by health care interpreters for most circumstances (Hatton and Webb 1993).

Strategies for interpretation between languages

Interpretation is part of the communication with which all nurses should be concerned regardless of their own or their patient's linguistic abilities. However, there are clearly particular issues when faced with a patient who speaks little or no English. This last section considers the options currently available:

- a nurse can 'make do', relying on mime and guesswork;
- the patient's family members or friends can interpret;
- staff who are not clinically qualified can be used as interpreters;
- clinically qualified staff who happen also to be bilingual can be called upon;
- a trained medical interpreter (not a clinician) or a link-worker may be employed;
- a telephone interpretation service can be used;
- the nurse may herself speak the patient's language fluently.

The main constraint on options for interpretation is the resources made available for interpretation by nurses' employers.

Inadequate strategies continue to be used because there is insufficient provision for interpretation in healthcare settings.

Making do

Some communication is possible if the professional is prepared to use every cue available, including the non-verbal cues. A nurse should never assume that a patient has no useful language skills. If a patient has arrived at a non-emergency consultation, unaccompanied by translator, they may well have some English language ability and some basic steps can be taken to maximize its utility (Henley 1991). A person may understand more than they can speak, so a lack of response from a patient does not necessarily mean they understand nothing. Incorporating advice for communicating with patients who have limited English in health care delivery to all patients, regardless of their linguistic fluency, would improve the transparency of communication with English speakers too.

Patient's friends or family members

When a patient knows that their spoken English is inadequate for health encounters, they are likely to be accompanied by a friend or relative with greater ability. In the absence of any other form of interpreter, this is of obvious benefit to both service user and provider. A friend or family member may be able to fulfil the role of advocate for the patient more effectively than a stranger because of their greater familiarity. However, there are two major pitfalls. First, the interpreter may withhold information from the patient or from the clinician for a number of reasons. The relative may wish to protect the patient from knowledge of the gravity of their illness (Vu 1996), or a paternalistic desire to safeguard the patient may mean that the interpreter feels they are best qualified to judge what lies in her best interests (Brafman 1995). For reasons of modesty or embarrassment men and women may feel unable to mention some conditions or areas of the body in one another's presence (Haffner 1992). Whatever the reason for the interpreter withholding information, the result may be that the nurse is unable to gain the patient's understanding of and consent for their healthcare. Second, children may be used as interpreters, when emotionally and/or linguistically ill prepared, as starkly illustrated by the instance of a seven-year old being required to translate during her mother's prenatal ultrasound scan which showed that the unborn child had died in utero (Hatton and Webb 1993).

Non-clinical staff

Non-clinical bilingual staff in hospitals are routinely called upon to translate for patients. For instance security and cleaning staff were among those used in a South African psychiatric service (Drennan 1996). Despite having no special training, staff who happened to be bilingual in Australian and American hospital departments were responsible for the majority of all non-English language encounters (Baker *et al.* 1998; Stolk *et al.* 1998).

While non-clinical staff working in healthcare settings may have much to offer patients, they are nonetheless untrained in nursing, medicine, or interpretation, nor are they a trusted confidante chosen by the patient.

Clinically qualified staff

Some interpretation work may fall to bilingual hospital nurses because their work keeps them in constant contact with patients and other health professionals (Drennan 1996). While such nurses are uniquely well qualified to fulfil the more general role of cultural mediator and patient advocate, they are not trained for interpretation work, nor are they rewarded for undertaking it. Salaried hours that hospital nurses spend interpreting could be better used to pay for a professional interpreter, freeing up nurses to do nursing work (Rader 1988). There is a danger that minority ethnic nursing staff, who are assumed to have appropriate cultural and linguistic skills, are used to improve service delivery to patients of the same ethnic group. These staff should be consulted over such specialization in their careers and be rewarded for special skills they bring to the job (Gerrish *et al.* 1996).

Many hospitals do keep lists of clinical and non-clinical staff who are bilingual and prepared to be used as interpreters (Anonymous 1975; Mitchell *et al.* 1998), and while this is clearly better than nothing, it has not been subject to systematic evaluation against professional interpretation services.

Medical interpreter or link-worker

One survey found that at only 5 per cent of non-English language consultations was a trained interpreter employed (Hornberger *et al.* 1996). Translators are employed in some English language hospitals with a high proportion of non-English-speaking patients and advocacy may or may not be an explicit part of the worker's role (Haffner 1992; Hatton and Webb 1993; Baylav 1996).

The importance of trained translators is that they can offer expert interpretation of the language and culture of the patient to the health professional, but equally they can interpret the expectations and norms of the healthcare providers to the patient. The supportive role that a translator can fulfil may be therapeutic in itself. The possible equivalent disadvantage is that, given both patient and interpreter are likely to come from a local minority community, the patient might fear disclosure.

Medical interpreters are only employed where there is considerable need, so great demands are made on their time (Haffner 1992) and they are unlikely to be able to work outside office hours (Jones and Gill 1998). The range of languages that can be covered by a single person is limited, so interpreters will never be able to offer a universal translation service. The salary costs of a full-time interpreter prohibit poorer institutions and/or those with a smaller proportion of non-English speaking patients from employing a dedicated worker.

Remote interpreters – language lines

'Language lines' offer interpretation services over the telephone (Holmes 1990; Pointon 1996). The interpreter can translate simultaneously, if two handsets are available for nurse and patient, or consecutively, when a single handset is passed between the two interlocutors. Although interpreters themselves prefer to be present, the remote system is better than proximate interpretation in terms of more utterances on the part of the doctor and patient and fewer inaccuracies in translation (Hornberger *et al.* 1996).

'Language Line' services in Britain (http://www.language line.co.uk/index.htm) and the USA (http://www.languageline. com/) are available 24 hours per day and cover over 100 and 140 different languages respectively. The remote service offers better confidentiality because the interpreters are unlikely to come from the same locality as the patient (Jones and Gill 1998), and so may be suitable for the discussion of potentially stigmatizing matters. However, the lack of supportive interpersonal contact may make it unsuitable for the communication of complex or sensitive information (Jackson 1990). The Language Line service may mean the obligation to fund bilingual healthcare translators or link-workers will be avoided, although the two forms of interpretation do not need to be seen as mutually exclusive choices (Pointon 1996).

Bilingual nursing staff

Bilingual nursing staff is one solution to language barriers, although the need to interpret medical jargon and idiom for patients still applies. Bilingual hospital nurses may be used by other healthcare professionals as interpreters, but are also more likely to be able to call upon interpreters, compared to nurses working in the community. Given the difficulties of community nurses obtaining the services of trained interpreters (McCabe and Rocheron 1985), the benefits of learning the minority language of their patients are considerable (Wilson 1989). Even if nurses are only able to learn basic greetings, a limited ability to speak may be disproportionately important in ameliorating communication by putting patients at their ease.

Conclusion

Patients and nurses alike value skilled communication in the development of nurse–patient partnerships, but poor communication remains the major cause of complaints about healthcare. Much of this is attributable to a lack of resources, particularly time and staff, rather than a lack of expertise or motivation from healthcare professionals (Wilkinson 1998).

Communication between nurse and patient can be compromised in a number of ways, including speaking different languages, different varieties of the same language, employing different vocabularies or accents and holding different expectations of an encounter. The advocacy role adopted by nurses and the way that nurses work with trained interpreters and non-nurse advocates, depends on the wider view of appropriate professional roles. The role of advocate could certainly include more explicit reference to communication, particularly between speakers of different languages. However, before the nursing profession is able to make clear recommendations for interpretation services that would ameliorate their health service provision, a comprehensive national audit of existing services and how this compares with measured need for such services is necessary.

Useful guidelines have been formulated for nurses communicating across a language barrier (Henley 1991). Ideally the skills needed to work with an interpreter would be explicitly taught and assessed as an integral part of the nursing curriculum and as part of a broader effort to teach both effective communication and provision of healthcare across cultural as well as linguistic boundaries. Realistically, nurses and midwives who obtain the services of interpreters or advocates, usually have to work without any special training. The widespread absence of professional advocacy and interpretation services means that most nurses and midwives will have to make-do with their own and their patient's language skills and, despite the disadvantages, will have to use family members as interpreters. Guidelines

(Henley 1991) address working with professional interpreters and coping without one. In both instances, twice as much interview time as usual should be allowed. With professional interpreters, the nurse should schedule time to establish the terms of the interview with the interpreter before meeting the patient and should consult again once the patient has left to confirm a common understanding of the interview. The interpreter should be given a few minutes to initiate rapport with the patient prior to the nurse consultation. The nurse should try to confirm that patient and interpreter speak a mutually comprehensive language and establish whether any social differences or similarities exist that might jeopardize communication (age, gender, religion). Notes should be taken on the quality of communication and rapport.

Where the patient's relative or friend is the only available interpreter the nurse should try to establish the interpreter's relationship to the patient, since this might influence the information that the nurse seeks to elicit and communicate. In nonemergencies communication of sensitive or intimate information might be delayed until a professional interpreter can be found. The quality of the interpreter's spoken English should be considered since this might also affect what the nurse asks him/her to translate. Organizing a follow-up appointment with a professional interpreter or advocate would always be good practice. Children, as already stated, should not be used as interpreters, except in emergencies where there is no alternative, in which case their youth and their relationship to the patient must be taken into consideration.

When a nurse or midwife must offer health service without even a 'lay' interpreter available, this should be recorded in the notes and communicated to the nurse's manager. In this situation a nurse can optimize limited communication by speaking plain English, saying things in the right order, limiting information that has to be remembered and leaving the patient with a simple, legible written summary (Henley 1991).

7 Midwives and screening for haemoglobin disorders

Simon Dyson

Introduction

This chapter raises the issue of ethnicity in relation to selective screening for haemoglobin disorders such as sickle cell and beta-thalassaemia. The chapter begins with a description of sickle cell and thalassaemia, outlines some background to issues surrounding selective ante-natal screening for haemoglobin disorders, and reports on the problematic nature of ethnic categories apparently in use in effecting such selectivity. The chapter then examines possible pragmatic strategies available to healthcare workers, including taking cues about ethnicity of clients from skin colour, names, geographical origins, unspecified combinations of these three, from an imposition of the United Kingdom Census categories, or by asking the client. Each in turn is felt to present certain problems with regard to the haemoglobin disorders. A number of strategies are proposed. One is to document the social encounter whereby ethnic categorization is socially constructed by healthcare workers. Others include combining asking for clients' self-defined ethnicity in tandem with an open explanation of the haemoglobin disorder-specific reason for which the information is being sought.

Haemoglobin disorders

The haemoglobin disorders discussed here include the haemoglobinopathies, most notably haemoglobin S which in its homozygous state produces sickle cell anaemia, but also other variant haemoglobins such as haemoglobins C, D, E, and O Arab which in combination with haemoglobin S produce lesser but significant clinical symptoms. The haemoglobin disorders referred to here also include the thalassaemias, both alpha and beta-thalassaemia. In Britain the conditions and their respective carrier states are predominantly found in inner city districts, reflecting patterns of residence of minority ethnic communities (Balarajan and Raleigh 1993).

Sickle cell disorders are a group of serious inherited blood disorders the most common of which is sickle cell anaemia. This primarily, but not exclusively, affects people of African-Caribbean, Mediterranean, Middle-Eastern and Indian descent (Fleming 1982; Davies *et al.* 1993). Under certain conditions (low oxygen, stress, cold, dehydration) the red blood cells become hard, rigid and sickle-shaped causing excruciating to mild pain. These painful crises are the most common reason for sickle cell-related hospital admission in Britain (Brozovic and Anionwu 1984; Brozovic *et al.* 1987). Other complications may include overwhelming infections, sudden anaemia and chronic problems (strokes, blindness, renal failure, and mobility problems).

Beta-thalassaemia major is a condition where the red blood cells produced are almost empty of haemoglobin. It mainly, but once more not exclusively, affects those of Mediterranean, Middle Eastern, Pakistani and Indian descent (Davies *et al.* 1993). Without treatment the person would die in early childhood. The treatment for beta-thalassaemia is psychologically monotonous and time-consuming (Ratip *et al.* 1995), and may lead to non-compliance in adolescence (Angastiniotis *et al.* 1986). Current treatment involves monthly blood transfusions and injections of an iron-chelating agent (desferrioxamine) which is usually given sub-cutaneously using a syringe-driver pump over 10–12 hours between five and seven times a week. The only cure is a bone marrow transplant which remains a high risk procedure involving as it does the temporary destruction of the person's own bone marrow and hence their basic defences against opportunistic infections.

A range of authors have drawn attention to the apparent inequity of provision of screening, counselling, clinical and social services for sickle cell anaemia and beta-thalassaemia (World Health Organization 1988; Franklin 1988; National Association of Health Authorities and Trusts 1989; Anionwu 1991, 1993; Davies 1993; Davies *et al.* 1993; Atkin and Ahmad 1996; Atkin *et al.* 1998). At the same time there has been concern expressed that where differences between ethnic groups are expressed in terms of genetics it is likely that data will then be interpreted in a racist manner (Bradby 1996). There are already concerns about discrimination in employment (Draper 1991) and insurance (Nuffield Council on Bioethics 1993) on the basis of genetics. The challenge that the haemoglobin disorders present to practising midwives and nurses is that they return us to biological parentage, and potentially, therefore, to simplistic conceptions of 'race', the very conceptions that this book seeks to challenge.

Selective ante-natal screening for haemoglobin disorders

Considerations of ethnicity are vital in ante-natal screening for haemoglobin disorders, especially where the screening is selective not universal. Universal ante-natal screening is recommended by the Standing Medical Advisory Committee for areas with an ethnic minority antenatal population of over 15 per cent (Department of Health 1993a), and selective screening where the at risk ante-natal population is less than 15 per cent. Note that the emphasis is on the proportion of the *ante-natal* population not the overall population. At the 1991 Census ethnic minorities formed 6 per cent of the total population but 10 per cent of births were to minority ethnic groups, and owing to the younger age structure of many ethnic minority groups these proportions will be even greater by the 2001 Census. However, all health districts have populations at risk for sickle cell/thalassaemia and, even where proportions of minority ethnic groups are small, it is claimed that education of health professionals to undertake selective screening is cost-effective (Modell and Anionwu 1996; Zeuner *et al.* 1999).

Note that screening does not merely serve to identify and counsel carriers about their risk of a child with a major haemoglobin disorder. Where, on the basis of a screening question, clients are then given a blood test, this may identify a pregnant mother with full sickle cell anaemia not known to the services. Providing the best obstetric care for a mother with sickle cell anaemia has been shown to greatly improve birth outcomes (Smith *et al.* 1996). Those who carry the thalassaemia trait can be diagnosed in order to rule out confusion with iron deficiency and prevent damaging prescribing of unnecessary iron supplements (Modell and Modell 1990).

Where the overall proportion of ethnic minorities in the antenatal population is less than 15 per cent, and/or where testing for sickle cell and thalassaemia is carried out on a selective basis, a local policy is required on how to assess an individual's ethnic origin (Department of Health 1993a). The Standing Medical Advisory Committee on Sickle Cell, Thalassaemia and Other Haemoglobinopathies highlights the role of health professionals but midwives in particular (Department of Health 1993a: 32). A lack of knowledge on the part of midwives and obstetricians has been found to be a barrier to providing clients with information about ante-natal screening tests (Smith *et al.* 1994). Midwives' knowledge of the haemoglobin disorders is incomplete both in respect of knowledge of inheritance patterns and, significantly, in terms of which ethnic groups are potentially involved (Dyson *et al.* 1996a,b,c). In particular midwives tended to think that sickle cell could only affect peoples of African-Caribbean descent and that beta-thalassaemia could only affect those of Mediterranean descent.

It is not clear who makes the decision about allocation to ethnic category where selective screening takes place, but as will be argued, the problem runs deeper than merely requiring that the client is sensitively asked their perceived ethnicity in terms of the UK Census of Population categories. The Department of Health (1993a) claimed that the 1991 Census categories did not identify Italian, Greek and Turkish-Cypriot, or Middle-Eastern populations relevant to the haemoglobin disorders, and this remains a problem with the 2001 categories (see Aspinall 2000; and Johnson, this volume). At least in 1991 it was possible to use the full classification of 35 codes, which did permit an identification of North African, Arab, Iranian, Greek (including Greek Cypriot), and Turkish (including Turkish Cypriot) groups. However, Italian remained submerged within the 'Other European' category (Peach 1996b).

Hogg and Modell (1998) have developed estimates of carrier rates for different ethnic categories used in the 1991 Census. The categories have been modified to reflect the high carrier rates for thalassaemia among those of Cypriot and Italian

Table 7.1 Estimated haemoglobin disorder carrier rates for different ethnic groups.

1991 Census categories (slightly modified)	Estimated carrier rates for all haemoglobinopathies and thalassaemias %
White (excluding Cypriot and Italian)	0.1
Black-Caribbean	16.0
Black-African	25.0
Black-Other	16.0
Indian	4.3
Pakistani	4.5
Bangladeshi	7.3
Chinese	8.0
Other Asian	3.0
Other-Other	6.0
Cypriots	17.0
Italian	5.0

Source: Adapted from Hogg and Modell (1998).

descent who might otherwise be subsumed within the 'White' category.

There is no standard instrument currently used in laboratories to record ethnic origin (Davies *et al.* 2000), and a survey of current practice has found wide variations in the categories used for selective ante-natal screening (Bains and Chapman 1996). A complete list of the various categories used in ante-natal screening nationally includes those based on skin colour (black); on individual countries (Ghana, Nigeria, China); on generalized geographical areas (Mediterranean; South Asian; Caribbean); on continents (African); on discredited biological theories (Caucasian, race, of racial origin); on notions of departure from fixed biological races (mixed race); on colonial definitions of geography (East Indies); on combinations of skin colour and nationality (black British, white British); on combinations of skin colour and continent (black African); and on problematic definitions of opposites (non-North European) or catch-all categories (other Asian) where the assumptions underlying the naming system are not made clear. A number of these problems also exist in the 1991 Census categories (Anwar

1990), and the 2001 categories (Aspinall 2000). However, such widespread imprecision of thought suggests that there may coexist both inaccuracies in screening and racist treatment of clients.

However, what is actually required is a policy to assess people at risk for haemoglobin disorders (Modell and Anionwu 1996) and this is not quite the same thing as their ethnicity. It has been noted that the usefulness of ethnicity as an indicator of being at risk of a haemoglobin disorder will decline over time (Department of Health 1993a; Andrews *et al.* 1994).

Pragmatic responses

We need to consider how selective ethnicity for ante-natal haemoglobin disorder testing is determined 'on the ground', whether by midwives or by clerical staff. There are several possibilities.

First, there may be selectivity based on skin colour or facial characteristics. Karmi and Horton (1993) have noted the possibility that health professionals may use visible characteristics to allocate clients to ethnic groups. Indeed, midwives may be tempted to use this strategy of ethnic categorization by sight on the basis that 'it works'. There is after all a correlation (that is, an association but not a causal link) between black skin and likelihood of being a carrier for sickle cell (Smaje 1995a). Quite apart from the role such a strategy plays in perpetuating racist ideologies of biological hierarchies of races (James 1993; Bradby 1996) it rests on questionable assumptions, namely:

- Inherited characteristics which cannot be seen by the naked eye (such as variant haemoglobins) and visible variants (such as skin colour) are inherited independently of one another (Jones 1991). It is perfectly possible for someone who 'looks' white to carry the gene for sickle cell.
- We are being asked to utilize skin colour and facial features as a 'racialized' barrier. But different observers will draw boundaries between skin colours at different points. We will not then know which midwives are using which

particular cut-off point. Thus we cannot know whether we are classifying like with like when we put together observations from different individual midwives which go towards official monitoring statistics on ethnic origin. Perhaps this would matter less if 'common-sense' observation could be demonstrated to closely match clients' self-definitions. But we have evidence it does not. Observation of skin colour by interviewer was apparently tried in a 1983 General Household Survey in the UK and, apart from those of West Indian, Indian, Pakistani and Bangladeshi descent, 25 per cent of other minority ethnic groups including those of so-called mixed origin were recorded as white (Bulmer 1996).

Second, there may be selection strategies based on geo-graphical 'origin'. Country of birth is of course a confusion of ethnic identity with nationality (and once more may be experi-enced by the client as part of the racism which has required UK passports to be produced to obtain health services – Gordon and Newnham 1985). It is further complicated by the numbers born in the so-called 'New Commonwealth' who describe them-selves as 'white', amounting in the 1991 Census to 15 per cent of those born in India (Mason 1995; Peach 1996b). The U.K. Thalassaemia Society, the national self-help group for thalas-saemia, modify this geographical origin strategy in their poster 'Do you, your parents, or your grandparents come from . . . ?', a poster which shows shaded areas of Africa and Asia (U.K. Thalassaemia Society 1988). But this strategy probably already requires several generations to be added to the question for those of South Asian descent born in East Africa or the Caribbean. It is further subject to the problem that carrier status is liable to disassociate over time from current patterns in ethnic groups (Department of Health 1993a).

Third there may be discrimination derived from names. Hughes *et al.* (1996) are among those who have researched communities of South Asian descent by sampling on the basis of names. However, this does not identify those of African-Caribbean descent nor those who have changed names at mar-riage, nor those who may have had their names changed for them by immigration officials at the time of migration.

Fourth, there may be attempts at selectivity on the basis of a combination of such schemas. While replicating each of the faults identified above, this has the additional disadvantage of not distinguishing between selection strategies based on inclusion when *all* three approaches mark the client out as of minority ethnic status and inclusion when *any* one of the three techniques effects such a result.

Fifth, there may be the erroneous assumption that a client's responses to the categories used in the 2001 Census will resolve the issue. But the imposition of categories onto a respondent may mean irritation that pre set responses do not accord with the complexities of their self-identity. To take one example, many of Arab descent ticked the category 'White' in the 1991 Census (Al-Rasheed 1996), and may indeed do so again with the 2001 categories. Bulmer (1996) reports that the 1989 Census Test had a 0.5 per cent refusal because of the inclusion of a question on ethnicity and a further.7 per cent who objected to the ethnicity question. Clearly refusal is a possibility in antenatal screening. At least one district in the UK uses refusal to give ethnicity as a criterion for testing (Bains and Chapman 1996), despite guidelines that state that the right to refuse information about ethnicity must be respected and must not affect the service the client receives (Karmi and Horton 1993). Testing all those who refuse to supply their ethnic identity raises serious ethical questions and is contrary to some guidelines which emphasize the need for informed consent (Nuffield Council on Bioethics 1993). This is particularly the case in instances when the genetic information then provided proves to be unwanted (Stone and Stewart 1996).

Finally, asking for ethnicity on the basis of self-identification may capture some of the complexities of self-identity that naming systems miss. 'Anglo-Indian', 'Anglo-Italian' and 'Anglo-Iranian' are three examples the author received when conducting a community survey on knowledge of beta-thalassaemia (Dyson *et al.* 1993). Young people with haemoglobin disorders are themselves said to favour terms such as 'British Asian' (Bailey-Holgate 1996). However, and as the examples also suggest, self identifications, precisely because they draw upon concepts grounded in common sense, may themselves suffer from confusions of nationality and ethnicity, or from biological concepts of 'race'.

Healthcare researchers have been advised to collect as much information as possible (including ethnicity, country of birth, religion, language, and socio-economic status) and describe fully what they have done (McKenzie and Crowcroft 1996). Indeed in research it has been argued that a full and open explanation to the respondent of what one is interested in may maximise one's chances of being directed to the source of information most relevant to the research (Whyte 1984). Likewise, as Modell and Anionwu (1996: 141) suggest: 'If everyone is informed even when screening is selective, people have the opportunity of drawing attention to risk factors that might otherwise be overlooked, such as the existence of a parent or grandparent from a risk group'.

An appropriate strategy would therefore seem to be to guide the client to that aspect of ethnicity relevant to the haemoglobin disorders and to gain thereby not an unproblematic 'true' allocation to an ethnic category, but a socially negotiated estimate of the likelihood of the client being a carrier for a haemoglobin disorder.

Using census categories may not accord with respondents' self identity, and in particular with the situational, dynamic and complex nature of that identity. It may leave a small number untested who describe themselves as 'white' (for example those of Mediterranean or Arab descent or those who choose this category above others to which they feel they might equally belong) given the untheorized nature of this category (Bradby 1995). It also means compounding the ethical issues of screening further when refusals are taken to be indicative of an ethnicity of likely disproportionate relevance to haemoglobin disorders.

The social construction of ethnicity

Through detailed observational ethnographic research, sociologists have drawn attention to the way in which policy and practice in organizations frequently does not occur in the way it is 'supposed to'. This suggests that we need to consider what actually happens (rather than what is supposed to or what is claimed to happen) and how the midwife and her client both help to *create* the meaning of ethnicity through their interaction (see Porter (1998) for the background to the ideas of symbolic interactionism).

Both predetermined categories and self-identification ignore the social encounter within which the information is asked. For example, who asks? of whom? at what time? with what demeanour? with what words? with what supplementary explanations as to the use of the information? is the given answer the one accepted? and so on. These ideas are elaborated below.

In terms of who asks, there are the prior questions of whether a record of ethnicity has been made in primary health care as Pringle and Rothera (1996) have suggested is possible and/or whether the inquirer is a clerk or a health care professional such as a midwife. There is then the issue of the ethnic characteristics of the inquirer. 'Race'-of-interviewer-effects have long been claimed in research interviews (Hyman 1954; Schuman and Converse 1971; Schaeffer 1980; Hagenaars and Heinen 1982) and DeLamater (1982) concludes that in so-called 'mixed race' pairings there is a tendency to avoid replies which are perceived as offending the other 'race'. But what subtle interactional clues do midwives and mothers give one another in 'sizing up' each other's ethnicity? And do these interactions themselves change the ethnic identity which midwives and mothers ascribe both to each other and the one they ascribe to themselves? More recent studies (Rhodes 1994) suggest that the response of black people to white interviewers and black interviewers are not more or less truthful, merely different. We do not yet know what different responses to haemoglobin disorders may be constructed by different ethnicities of the inquirer. However, we do know that the quality of the encounter from the point of view of the ethnic minority client seems improved if they feel that the haemoglobinopathy counsellor is of the same ethnic group as themselves (Anionwu 1996). Indeed some haemoglobinopathy counsellor posts may represent the few occasions in nursing where bilingual skills are recognized in job descriptions and reflected in the seniority of the grade.

Equally important given the particular minority ethnic groups affected by haemoglobin disorders in the UK is the language in which the exchange takes place (Rehman and Walker 1995). On the basis of UK research (Rudat 1994), and utilizing the most appropriate sub-category, namely that of women aged 16–29, it appears that 49 per cent of Indian descent; 63 per cent of Pakistani descent and 86 per cent of Bangladeshi descent *do not* consider English to be their main language. The quality of the haemoglobin-specific information on ethnicity that is given and received therefore also depends upon the availability of high quality interpreting services or on bilingual health workers (Anionwu 1996). However, ethnic minority patients report that use of informal interpreters in health settings apparently still exceeds formal interpreting provision (Rudat 1994: 66).

There are issues too concerning whether questions on ethnicity are selectively asked. Pringle and Rothera (1996) report that health staff and receptionists in an area of the UK with a low prevalence of minority ethnic groups felt far more uncomfortable in asking patients their ethnicity than did their counterparts in an area of high minority ethnic group presence. Might white midwives or clerical staff with little experience of relating to minority ethnic groups find strategies to avoid asking the client their ethnicity directly, perhaps because they fear offending them? This suggests the importance of appropriate training being provided for all health workers involved in asking or encoding ethnic data (Karmi and Horton 1993).

Social context in time is also of relevance to any exchange asking about ethnicity. Bulmer (1996) records how local campaigns against the 1979 UK Census Test based on claims that the information would be linked to proposed changes in the nationality law (eventually the 1981 British Nationality Act, which removed the automatic right of all people born on British soil to British citizenship) led to non-responses by almost half the households and led the Office of Population, Censuses and Surveys (OPCS) to conclude that an ethnicity question in the 1981 Census would not be successful. Although the question was asked in the 1991 UK Census, one reason for under enumeration was the fear that the data would be linked to poll tax registers then kept by local authorities for the purposes of local taxation. Under enumeration was a feature of young inner city residents and both these factors would over represent minority ethnic groups in the shortfall. There is no reason to suppose that more local collection of ethnic data would not also be affected by national or indeed local political contexts.

Finally, there is the social orientation of the health worker to the client. In ante-natal screening this will most frequently be the midwife and the mother. To the extent that some midwives do, as Bowler (1993a,b) claims, racially stereotype mothers of South Asian descent this will compromise the quality of a conversation attempting to establish ethnicity.

Thus overall the social context may crucially affect, if not the validity of the reply (for that would be to falsely assume that there exists one 'true' answer) then the authenticity of the reply (by which is meant the extent of any intention on the part of the respondent to deliberately mislead or to withhold information). A description of such encounters would be a first step in establishing the difficult question as to how we should advise health professionals to conduct screening for haemoglobin disorders in the absence of universal screening.

Achieving selectivity in screening

Notwithstanding the complexities of the arguments discussed here, the fact remains that many areas of the UK will continue to operate selective ante-natal screening for haemoglobin disorders for the foreseeable future. What might constitute a way forward where midwives are faced with decisions about whether to screen at all, and sometimes how to screen selectively?

Localized universal screening involves taking policy decisions about whether the local ethnic composition merits universal haemoglobin disorder screening. This assumes that relevant ethnic communities are enumerated in official statistics to enable decisions based on thresholds to take place. The UK is in a small minority of Western European countries in asking a Census question on ethnicity (as distinct from citizenship, religion, or language) (Coleman and Salt 1996b), and it is the availability of such data which permits the Department of Health (1993a) to put forward its recommendation of a threshold of a 15 per cent ethnic minority ante-natal population to trigger ante-natal sickle cell screening. Such localized universal screening implies that, irrespective of the cut-off points used, certain districts will continue to screen only selectively. The question still remains therefore of how to effect such selectivity. The following are some tentative suggestions on how this might be achieved at ante-natal clinics.

● An increase in the number of haemoglobinopathy nurse counsellors permits education of midwives, nurses and health service interpreters/advocates on haemoglobin disorders. The educational programmes should also include the views of those living with sickle cell anaemia or beta-thalassaemia.

● A midwife trained in this way can then explain to the mother the existence and the basic clinical symptoms of the relevant haemoglobin disorder(s). This explanation should be in the client's first language and will depend upon employment of bilingual health workers or health interpreters and advocates (see Bradby, this volume, and Anionwu 1996). The midwife can explain that the haemoglobin disorders are inherited, and that carrier states can be detected through a blood test. The carrier state offers in some cases protection against certain types of malaria in childhood and is therefore associated with populations who live in areas of the world where malaria is, or was, prevalent, and with their descendants. The variant haemoglobins are passed through generations without carriers necessarily being aware of their status.

● The client is asked if they are aware of any ancestors, however many generations removed, who may have originated in key areas of the world. Schott and Henley (1996) suggest that the midwife needs to know any special terms for referring to grandparents on the father's or mother's side. The client could be prompted with a look-up table based on the Regional Tables of Annex 1 of the *Guidelines for the control of haemoglobin disorders* (World Health Organization 1994) which give estimates of carriers of each relevant variant haemoglobin for each country or by permitting the client to point to a map of the world (Department of Health 1993a). On the basis of this discussion the client is asked to describe their own ethnicity, using more than one descriptor if so wished. In order that some aggregation is facilitated (because this more detailed information may in turn inform policy decisions about thresholds for screening) it is suggested that the full 35 ethnic codes of the 1991 Census be used (Peach 1996a) (or their equivalents in 2001) with appropriate descriptors where necessary (e.g. to further describe 'Other Asian' and 'Any Other White background').

● The midwife explains the processes of screening and testing and the potential range of results, outlining the potential uses to which information may be put. This may include clinical uses for the mother herself (diagnosis of sickle cell disorder or the carrier state for sickle cell or drawing a distinction between iron deficiency and being a carrier for beta-thalassaemia). Or it may involve information relating to reproductive choices (initiating a test of the father; the possibility of testing the foetus in utero if both parents are found to be carriers, for example). As part of the screening question, the mother can then be asked *whether she wishes to be tested*: an essential feature of the guidance of the Nuffield Council on Bioethics (1993).

There are legitimate questions about whether testing should proceed if there is no identified purpose. The mother may not wish to consider a termination under any circumstances. She may not find advance warning of a child with a major haemoglobin disorder useful. She may not wish to have the responsibility of informing the rest of the family, including her children, of the increased possibility that they are carriers. The range of controversial issues indicated here is extensive. Rothman (1994) has pointed out that genetic information places mothers in moral dilemmas not of their own choosing and could be said to decrease rather than increase women's choice. Attitudes, not only to termination, but also to whether to accept the medical discourse of genetic inheritance at all have been shown to relate to socio-economic position and the symbolic importance of children to African-American women living in poverty (Hill 1994). The variability of sickle cell disorders has been shown to mitigate against termination (Anionwu *et al.* 1988), the course of beta-thalassaemia being more predictable. Davies *et al.* (2000) suggest that 80 per cent of beta-thalassaemia major and 16 per cent of sickle cell anaemia births are prevented by ante-natal screening. This suggests that an explanation of the nature of the relevant conditions be part of the pre-testing counselling. This will inevitably involve extra resources, both in training of counsellors and in ongoing execution of the tasks. The counselling raises further issues concerning the extent to which non-directive counselling is possible (Clarke 1991) and indeed whether the thought of imposing the costs of treating a child with a genetic disorder onto the parents might one day be raised (Clarke *et al.* 1992). Pre-screening counselling may appear to be an expensive option in health economic terms. However, there are several arguments against such a rejection on the basis of cost.

It is considered vital that those pregnant women offered an HIV-antibody test ante-natally are counselled because of the potentially devastating impact of the test results on that person and their significant others (Department of Health 1993b). Genetic information associated with the haemoglobin disorders is surely no less important.

To the extent that failure to screen or to warn of a genetic disorder, or alternatively subjecting clients to unwanted screening interventions, may result in litigation, costs to health-care providers might be reduced by sensitive pre-screening counselling.

To the extent that successful community education programmes are carried out, this may in turn reduce the time required for counselling explanations (Modell *et al.* 1991). Indeed successful community education could result in greater levels of pre-conceptual and solicited requests for screening, broaden the responsibility to men and reduce the need for potentially distressing information to be raised for the first time in early pregnancy. If everyone is informed about the screening process then clients are enabled to draw attention to factors such as having a relative from an at-risk group (Modell and Anionwu

1996). In primary care, Modell *et al.* (1998) show that practice nurses can be willing to undertake pre-conceptual carrier screening.

If one accepts the argument that quality of information given to the client will improve quality of information emanating in turn from the client, cases where a child is born with a major haemoglobin disorders may be reduced. Indeed, in one study of collecting ethnic data in general practice nearly half of patients felt that a 'specially trained person' should ask about their ethnicity (Pringle and Rothera 1996).

This brings us to the moral issue of selective termination on the rights and images of people with disabilities. Hogg and Modell (1998) propose that pre-screening information can reduce anxieties in clients and help people prepare for the potential results of testing. But any description of what the life of someone with sickle cell or thalassaemia is like will involve moral judgements about the potential lives of people living with sickle cell anaemia or thalassaemia. The phrasing of a recent Health Technology Assessment Report (Davies *et al.* 2000) raises issues about the rights of those living with sickle cell/thalassaemia, because of the way they are described in health economics terms. In this description the economic viability of ante-natal screening for sickle cell is explicitly linked to the lower uptake of terminations than is the case for beta-thalassaemia. To be fair, Davies *et al.* (2000) also mention the importance of genetic choice as an outcome measure of screening, but this does raise questions about the way in which people living with sickle cell anaemia/beta-thalassaemia major are described by midwives in giving explanations of the conditions to clients (see Dyson 1999).

While it is undoubtedly true that genetic counselling could be subverted into pressures to abort to meet public health goals (Harper 1992), more positive potential exists. Forms of questioning in counselling exist which open spaces to 'preferred realities' in opposition to questioning which accepts uncritically problem-saturated accounts (Freedman and Coombs 1996), including perhaps problem-saturated accounts of the potential lives of children with chronic illness. In the context of narrative therapy, White and Epston (1990) record the development of community groups or leagues with databases consisting of successful stories of living with a variety of challenging conditions, experiences or circumstances which act as a resource for the respective communities of interest. The establishment of such databases for the haemoglobin disorders, while themselves having the potential to be invoked in oppressive ways (if successful life stories create automatic moral expectations that people should cope with their circumstances) does offer the possibility of counterbalancing prevailing genetic discourses which ultimately carry assumptions of saving on the costs of treating those with haemoglobin disorders (Ostrowsky *et al.* 1985; Angastiniotis *et al.* 1986; World Health Organization 1988; Zeuner *et al.* 1999; Davies *et al.* 2000). Pre-screening counselling could thereby constitute a modest accentuation of the choices available to the mother in opposition to the screening-prenatal diagnosis-termination assumptions which appear at present to be dominant in the experiences of women at antenatal clinics (Rothman 1994).

Conclusion

This chapter has sought to draw attention to the problematic relationship between genetic screening policies and ethnic minorities in the UK. Where universal screening for haemoglobin disorders takes place, the dangers are that clients are not informed of the specific tests to which their blood is to be subjected; are not given explanations of the haemoglobin disorders themselves until a person is identified as a carrier, and may not be asked whether or not they even wish to be tested. These dilemmas also arise where selective testing occurs, but to these are added the problems of how precisely ethnic identity is established; the adequacy of the knowledge base of the person describing the client's ethnicity; and above all the dilemmas of the different ways of classifying ethnicity, each of which fails to capture the aspects of ethnicity relevant for selective ante-natal screening for sickle cell/thalassaemia.

The areas where practice might be improved include the ethics of establishing prior informed permission to test; the sensitive establishing of ethnicity, not merely through blanket categories, but geared to the specific health purpose for which the information is sought; determining who wishes for information; the provision of information; the provision of accurate information; and the provision of information within a discourse which accentuates a range of possibilities rather than a discourse which effectively determines outcomes under the guise of choices.

A possible strategy, though not without cost implications, has been identified as one which involves a considered taking of client histories in which explanations of haemoglobin disorders are linked to clients' perceptions of their ethnicity given in the light of this information. Such histories may usefully be guided by World Health Organization estimates of carrier rates worldwide. Some information for local targeting of community education and for national comparisons might be provided by use of expanded census categories as well as open-ended responses to the question of ethnicity.

Such a professional–client encounter could also constitute a pre-screening counselling session, which, as with HIV antibody testing, helps determine whether the information and/or testing is relevant to the client's expressed needs. In this way unwanted and inappropriate testing can be avoided, and the testing that does proceed is based on consent, and on *informed* consent, and on consent which has been given an opportunity to consider the import of the screening process in the context of individual life histories and socio-cultural situations.

However, the socio-cultural context is open to particular representations by the health professional, who in reporting on genuine perceptions of the very real challenges of poverty, a gender ordered society, racisms and discriminations against people with disabilities, may, in their very desire to protect the client from such challenges, not be aware of or fail to reveal to the client, those occasions, circumstances and people whose lives contain real elements of enjoyment and success. Community leagues or databases of such success stories, preferably controlled by patient self-help groups or others beyond the health professionals themselves, could function as a resource which could counterbalance what might otherwise be a dominant representation of living with sickle cell/thalassaemia as only being a negative experience.

The issue of midwives and selective ante-natal screening for the haemoglobin disorders suggests that while we need education about which ethnic groups are particularly affected, at the same time we need to understand that ethnicity is only an approximation of being a carrier for sickle cell/thalassaemia. Understanding this subtle distinction should help improve practice in terms not only of the screening itself but also in terms of developing better informed consent and community education. Furthermore, considerations of ethnicity are rarely able to be taken in isolation of other inequalities such as gender and disability (see Dyson 1999), which also require attention in order to promote best practice. Finally, if, as seems likely, screening for haemoglobin disorders is encouraged in primary care, then dilemmas of ethnicity and haemoglobin disorders will also become part of the work of practice nurses and health visitors.

8 Ethnicity and palliative care

Yasmin Gunaratnam

Introduction

Palliative care has been defined by the National Council for Hospice and Specialist Palliative Care Services (1995: 5) as the 'active total care of patients and their families by a multi-professional team when the patient's disease is no longer responsive to curative treatment'. In aiming to provide 'whole person' care, palliative care focuses upon physical symptom control as well as the psycho-social needs of the individual and their carer(s). It can be provided in a variety of settings including hospitals, hospices, residential and nursing homes, as well as in people's own homes.

In many ways, palliative care has transformed radically the care of dying people (James and Field 1992), reflecting a more person-centred approach than traditional medical models. However, there have also been growing concerns, in this country (Hill and Penso 1995; Field et al. 1997) and internationally (Brenner 1997; Waddell and McNamera 1997) about issues of cultural 'sensitivity'. In nursing practice, these concerns have been addressed largely within a culturalist framework, where education and training resources (for examples see Green 1989, 1992) have focused upon the need for nurses to be knowledgeable about the cultural and religious beliefs and practices of different groups. However, together with a growing awareness of the need for more complex approaches to ethnicity and culture, multicultural models, and more specifically, the culturalist elements that predominate within them, have been coming under increasing criticism (De Santis 1994; Culley 1996; Gunaratnam 1997). A basic fact remains that despite the implementation of a range of multicultural initiatives, many service users still experience forms of exclusion, both from, and within services. As a report into hospice and palliative care has noted, a fundamental anomaly is that '. . . despite the numerous guidelines that exist, it emerged that in nearly all cases services were provided in an ad hoc manner. The systems in place to achieve delivery of a culturally sensitive service were either unreliable or largely ineffective' (Hill and Penso 1995: 14).

In this chapter, I want to suggest that this gap between policy and practice is caught up with multicultural approaches themselves. In particular, what I will be examining, is how – within the context of work with dying people – multiculturalism can lead to particular forms of discrimination in which individuals can become dehumanized as 'others', so that differences serve to also construct false distances between 'us' and 'them' (Wilkinson and Kitzinger 1996). As Ien Ang (1996) has argued, within multiculturalism, '. . . racially and ethnically marked people are no longer othered today through simple mechanisms of rejection and exclusion, but through an ambivalent and apparently contradictory process of *inclusion by virtue of othering*' (p. 37; emphasis in original).

It is precisely because of these complex and often subtle processes of 'othering', that service provision and professional practice in this era of multiculturalism is characterized by uncertainty and dilemma. Rather than masking these difficult and 'messy' issues, I want to show how their recognition can be used to develop more responsive inter-cultural practice. In doing so, I want to first outline briefly the ways in which concerns about multiculturalism and 'race' equality have been framed within palliative care. I will then draw upon my qualitative research with service users and staff in a London hospice to explore three different, but interrelated aspects of service provision: by exploring what staff and service users say about the multicultural provision of food I will address examples of 'inclusion by virtue of othering'; I will then examine areas of insecurity in inter-cultural practice; and lastly I will address the way lived experiences of ethnicity and inequality have implications for holistic care.

A service development context: 'race' equality in palliative care

A general concern with equity in palliative care gained impetus in the 1990s in response to wider changes in the health service.

In particular, the introduction of a mixed economy of care following the National Health Service and Community Care Act 1990, has been identified as involving the 'heightened emphasis on consumer choice, on quality issues, cost-effectiveness and equity' (Clark 1994: 2). This somewhat broad concern, has been followed by increasingly more specific policy and service development directives, with guidance produced by the National Council for Hospice and Specialist Palliative Care Services in 1997 advising that:

> Setting formal standards is an opportunity to promote equal opportunities in employment and personnel practices, access to services and treatment of patients/carers. Standards should recognise diversity of religion, culture and language in the populations served. (Glickman 1997: 20)

Although these statements engage with particular aspects of diversity, in common with other statements on equity in the health service, they are still 'notoriously ambiguous' (O'Donnell and Popper 1991: 2). Nevertheless, what is notable is how concerns about ethnic diversity have been largely interpreted in relation to service access, use and acceptability. Indeed such concerns were most forcefully articulated in 1995, with the publication of the report *Opening Doors*, by the National Council for Hospice and Specialist Palliative Care Services (Hill and Penso 1995). The report included the findings of research carried out into hospice and palliative care provision to 'black and Asian' people with cancer in Brent, Newham, and Birmingham Health Authorities. The report based its definitions of 'black' and 'Asian' on the 1991 Census categories of ethnicity. As such the category 'black' was used to refer to people who classified themselves as 'Black Caribbean', 'Black African' and 'Black Other'. The term 'Asian' was used to refer to people who classified themselves as 'Indian', 'Pakistani' and 'Bangladeshi'. The report chose to focus upon people with cancer since, 'The majority of the people receiving hospice care are people with cancer' (p. 8).

In addressing access and the use and acceptability of services, the report echoed many of the concerns of wider debates on ethnicity and health service provision, highlighting two central issues. First, there was the belief that black and Asian people had not been provided with fair access to services, and were therefore under-represented among users of the services. Second, there was the concern that existing provision was not meeting their needs.

While the lack of accurate data on the ethnicity of service users in the study localities made it difficult for the research to determine the under-use of services, the report identified several factors that were seen as contributing to the perceived low take up of services. These factors included, the relatively lower incidence of cancer within black and Asian populations (Balarajan and Bulusu 1990); and the fact that deaths from cancer occur mainly in people over 55 years of age. The relatively younger age structures of black and Asian populations, together with the researchers' contention that 'many' older people 'emigrate back to their country of origin in later life' (p. 15), were seen as possible explanations for the perceived low take-up of services.

With regard to the acceptability of service provision, the study examined interviews with hospital and hospice staff, suggesting that a mixture of both structural service provision and attitudinal factors were affecting the acceptability of services. These factors included the 'ad hoc' provision of interpreting services; inadequate dietary provision; a lack of facilities to meet a diversity of religious and cultural needs; and the low numbers of 'black and Asian' doctors, nurses and related health and palliative care professionals.

Of course many of these factors are not 'new' and reflect more general inadequacies in health service provision that have been noted by a number of different researchers (Ahmad 1993; Baxter 1989; Swarup 1993). However, it is also the case that equitable service provision is more complex and problematic than such analyses suggest. Indeed, what I want to suggest is that concerns about service accessibility, utilisation and acceptability can serve to distort and simplify lived experiences of ethnicity, inequality and of inter-cultural relations. As Ahmad (1993) has suggested, health services often misrepresent the complex nature of service inequalities through a preoccupation with cultural differences in shaping the service experiences of different ethnic groups. Moreover, within palliative care there are also relatively little data that 'inform an understanding of the context within which people from minority ethnic groups may use palliative care services, and their views and experiences of service provision' (Smaje and Field 1997: 142).

In putting forward a case for the rethinking of inter-cultural service provision, I will be suggesting that we need to move away from some of the common-sense certainties that have marked traditional service initiatives and move towards more flexible, but necessarily incomplete and temporary *processes* of service development. With increasingly complex and changing forms of ethnic and cultural identification, it is simply not enough to address the needs of service users through the same basic multicultural initiatives that have been with us for more than 20 years. Bauman (1996) has suggested, that when the rules of one's 'life-game' keep changing according to constantly moving identities, 'The sensible strategy is therefore to keep each game short' (p. 24). Similarly, many multicultural approaches need to be 'kept short' and evaluated continually in the light of changing experiences of ethnicity and of inequality. These issues will be addressed in more detail in the following sections where I look at the multicultural provision of food, professional practice and holistic care.

Food for thought

In looking at the multicultural provision of a range of food options for service users, what I want to explore are the ways this seemingly inclusive provision can be based upon contradictory and oversimplified notions of ethnicity and culture. This is not to deny the importance of the availability of a range of food for service users, or to deny the links between ethnicity, culture, religion and food. The main difficulty is that such 'special needs' provision is structured to function around rationalistic associations based upon fixed categories of ethnicity and 'need'. Precisely because of the advantages of the administrative neatness of these associations, the 'messiness' of lived experiences – for people of all ethnicities – can be excluded from consideration.

For instance, in this contemporary period, marked by increasingly complex forms of migration and globalization, it is possible to see quite vividly how different cultural forms are continually evolving and changing. Many individuals are able to experiment or 'play' with aspects from different cultures such as with food, music or clothes, that can in turn lead to the creation or synthesis of new cultural forms. Such cultural interdependencies are creating a variety of forms of living and choices for all service users which remain unrecognized within multicultural approaches. Moreover, choices about food can also be seen as involving sensuality and pleasure (how food looks, smells, tastes and feels). However, modern bureaucratic service provision tends to deal poorly with such experiences (Mellor and Shilling 1997), with the emphasis frequently being on the economic management and disciplining of choices. Institutions therefore often have to look for the lowest common denominator of 'choice', and produce a fixed range of options in attempts to manage diversity. In this context, culturalist approaches that offer seemingly straightforward links between ethnicity, culture, religion and food can appear to provide a useful way of addressing differences in need. The difficulty is that this rationalistic approach to food can serve to obscure the complex relations between cultural identifications and food choices, whilst also failing to recognize the modifications to particular constructions of 'cultural' diets that some service users may wish/need to make as a result of changing experiences of disease and illness.

The unique nature of such relations has implications for how variations in experiences of culture, religion, sensuality and disease can make a difference to the relevance of the provision of different types of food to service users. At a practical level this also means that it can be particularly difficult to monitor and evaluate the effectiveness of certain provisions by traditional measures. For instance, during my research, the hospice had formalized its commitment to the provision of multicultural food options for 'in-patients'. As a part of this commitment, dietary choices were to be addressed during the admissions process. Yet, several weeks after implementation, concerns were raised because of the apparent low uptake of the 'ethnic' food options. In looking at my interviews with service users, it was possible to see that a complex inter-lacing of idiosyncratic and culturally related elements were frequently involved in the choices that people made, serving to destabilize any predictable relationships between ethnicity, culture, religion and food. Issues of cultural sensitivity, and most significantly relations of exclusion, then become not only more ambiguous and uncertain, making them difficult to monitor, they also become highly political.

The area of religious prescription, where relations with food are typically seen as more stable, provides an illustration of these ambiguous processes. I spoke to two Muslim service users and a carer, all of whom used different strategies to negotiate dimensions of individual preference, religious prescription and perceptions of the quality of the food provided by the hospice. A Pakistani woman, a lone parent, without relatives in this country, said that when in the hospice she chose the vegetarian option because she rarely ate meat and also liked to have English food. The carer told me that her husband who was Pakistani, had chosen the Kosher food because he could not tolerate spicy food at that stage of his illness, although she also added that she felt he did not like the halal food, speculating that it was probably cooked using curry paste and not raw spices. A Bangladeshi man told me that his wife, or brother-in-law always brought him home-cooked food, because the halal food in the hospice was 'completely bad'. In common with other service users, he doubted that the hospice could ever provide him with food that could meet his individual preferences.

Some of these experiences can be more easily interpreted as responses to cultural insensitivity in service provision, for instance the choice of Kosher food, in part because of the method of cooking halal food, using paste rather than raw spices. However, others are more porous, reflecting not simply the inappropriateness of provision, but also variations in individual preferences, and the wider social context of peoples lives, such as the availability of alternative forms of provision and care, and gender relations. Yet, the extent to which these experiences can be seen to fall within the concerns of multiculturalism, particularly when viewed in relation to the experiences of white, English service users is extremely problematic. For example, a nursing auxiliary in a discussion about caring observed that 'We've got a chap on the ward at the moment, he's English and his Gran brings him in pie and mash. He loves pie and mash, and maybe three times week he has his pie and mash . . . or pie and liquor'.

What this example illustrates is a common omission within multiculturalism, that is how cultural experiences of English-ness also have implications for service provision. In broad terms, the choices of many white, English people are also not met by services and some of these choices may relate to cultural experiences of age, class and region. For both English and non-English service users then, there are practical limitations in providing for a diversity of choices. However, through the association of multiculturalism with 'exotic' differences largely based upon differences of colour, ethnicity, culture and religion, the experiences of minority ethnic people can become marginalised, not simply through processes of exclusion but also through more subtle processes of inclusion. At the same time, the experiences of the ethnic majority are seen to fall outside the concerns of multiculturalism, so that experiences of 'whiteness' or 'Englishness' are seen as unproblematic and one-dimensional.

Which experiences are addressed, how, and through what mechanisms, then inevitably involves difficult political decisions, through which fundamental judgements are made that have repercussions for the representation and understanding of ethnicity, multiculturalism and of service use. Traditional multicultural initiatives, such as those relating to food, are based upon the important recognition that a diversity of service options are important in providing symbolic and practical respect and a valuing of the differences between service users (Gerrish *et al.* 1996). What I am suggesting is that these same approaches can also often be based upon a distortion of experiences that in sometimes paradoxical ways, can actually maintain and sometimes increase the perceived differences, and also distances between 'us' and 'them'. So in some cases multiculturalism can lead to the exclusion of a diversity of experiences, reflecting an anxious and tokenistic service provision, that at best is able to address a limited range of experiences. In hospitals, food provision is liable to be even more bureaucratically organized than in hospices. In such circumstances nurses are best advised to offer the full range of menu options to the patient rather than assume their needs on the basis of their presumed ethnicity. Once again, nursing in an appropriate manner involves being open to negotiating with the client their dietary and other needs (see Chapter 5, this volume).

Insecure practice

Having looked at some of the ways in which some multicultural service initiatives can lead to the distortion of manifestations of ethnicity and culture, I want to explore the relations between representations of professional practice and ethnic and cultural difference. During my research, I facilitated 14 group interviews with 38 members of hospice staff. Within our discussions, I found that inter-cultural work was frequently identified with levels of anxiety, characterized by feelings of fear, uncertainty and ambivalence. Although these feelings can arise in a variety of services, the very nature of palliative care work appeared to generate specific material, emotional and symbolic environments for staff that were seen as affecting inter-cultural work. As one member of staff said:

> I was thinking why it is so frightening and I think it is about communication, particularly around death. In our own culture it is difficult, even when there are already agreed concepts and understanding around death, but when you are dealing with people from another culture, you are adding another layer. You have already trebled the difficulty if you like. You don't know if you are using the right words, and even if you do speak the same language the depth of understanding of the other person's culture is very shallow on one side ... in the context of dying we often have to reach out to people and take risks, and I think I might be more reluctant to do that with people from a different culture.

In the latter part of this extract, the speaker makes links between feelings of fear and reticence and the impact these have upon his practice, in particular, his reluctance to 'take risks'. While there can be little doubt that some palliative care staff engage in very direct forms of discrimination, I found that processes of 'othering' could also involve inaction or the restriction of practice, such as a failure to take potentially creative risks with practice (Gunaratnam *et al.* 1998). For instance, some of the most enabling and creative work that staff do frequently involves boundary testing and risk taking – such as acting upon intuitive hunches, challenging themselves or service users, trying something new or different. Yet, as this next interview extract indicates, when some staff examined aspects of their inter-cultural work, feelings of uncertainty and fear were talked about as inhibiting these more creative aspects of their practice:

> I was thinking of a . . . black family and . . . the mother who's ill . . . and she's very closed down . . . and everything is in her head . . . I don't think that I challenged that in her. I couldn't take the risk . . . I feel very aware . . . around black, Afro-Caribbean culture, around respect being very, very important as well as not being clear about the rules and boundaries and the cultural etiquettes around that. But I wonder if that's also me being frightened of actually saying 'Looking X., you're very pragmatic. You're very philosophical, but I actually don't believe that you aren't sad about the prospect that you are going to die and you're not worried about your son' . . . so I do wonder if I would have been different with a white person.

Other significant themes in talk about inter-cultural work related to feelings of ambivalence and the construction of dilemmas for practice. Hence, many individuals talked about inter-cultural work in terms of powerful feelings of either 'getting it right' or 'getting it wrong', others deliberated about the validity of their perceptions of cultural phenomena, while others talked about the difficulties of managing inter-cultural differences between service users (Gunaratnam 1997). The issue here is not that staff were unable to respond to difference, but that they often did so with feelings of uncertainty and ambivalence. This uncertainty can be heard in the following extract from a group discussion with nurses, which begins with Gill considering whether her inability to communicate with an African service user was because of ethnic and cultural differences:

> *Gill*: I was just thinking about this one lady in particular, I found it extremely hard to get alongside her, I would say because of the cultural differences . . . I'm not sure, there was a lot to her case in particular . . . but I found it with Ugandan women in particular actually, that I find it very difficult to, to I suppose read them. You know, I suppose I go a lot on peoples' non-verbals as well as what they say, and when the language is different you go a lot on peoples' non-verbals . . . so it was very difficult, but I found we never really got alongside her . . . I suppose I view that as a failure of care in a way. . . . but then can you, can we ever, as somebody from a different culture . . . could I ever have done that given more time? . . . So you know I don't really know . . .
>
> *Roz*: . . . yes . . . if that was me, as a nurse I would be really worrying that I hadn't done my best by that person . . . and was it . . . because I

was white and hadn't a clue about her background? Whether that was what held me up?

Kate: Yeah, but some patients . . . wherever they're from. . . .

Roz: Yeah, are really private.

Kate: Go in on themselves when they're dying and have to find . . . the strength from within, which means they don't speak . . .

Roz: I think it's a feeling that you might have failed them . . . that for me is quite hard, 'cause I think "well, as a nurse I'm here 'cause I want to be useful and if somebody is very private then you can't be . . . So is that me having a problem because I haven't achieved, 'cause I want the sort of kick I want to get out of nursing?" Or has indeed that person missed out on something that, that they would have found useful? Or that in other circumstances, with other people they would have accessed? . . .

Within this extract is a mixture of issues that reach beyond simplistic binaries of 'good' or 'bad' practice. What is significant about this case is the nurses' uncertainty about any of the consequences of cultural difference, that despite their speculations can never actually be verified, leaving many questions raised but unanswerable. Interestingly, such questions also appear to be intertwined with representations of nursing, that serve to further intensify the nature of the deliberations. Indeed, the reality of much inter-cultural practice, is that it is often fragmentary and ambiguous, in which some experiences can be addressed, while others can be misrepresented, suppressed or excluded from consideration. What is a cause of concern is not that these ambiguities can characterise professional practice, but that they can often be pathologized by multicultural approaches that emphasize the harmonious and unproblematic nature of work, making it difficult for practitioners to address openly some of the difficulties of inter-cultural relations. Thus, although Gill framed the distances between herself and the African woman as a 'failure of care', her feelings of uncertainty can also be seen more positively as evidence of an awareness of some of the complexities and ambiguities of inter-cultural work that have been largely ignored within multiculturalism.

In opposition to the rationale behind many multicultural approaches, I would suggest that recognition of the 'messiness' and complexities of inter-cultural work can actually be productive for some staff, serving to exorcise rigid and moralistic notions of 'correctness' that are often associated with inter-cultural and anti-discriminatory practice. As one person described, formal commitments to multiculturalism and equal opportunities can sometimes actually make it more difficult for staff to explore and to ask for help around areas of ambiguity in practice, because

> ... it would be a bit like identifying yourself as having racist tenden-cies. I think all the drive against racism in organisations has some-times also been counterproductive and has pushed it underground. Racist people are more circumspect now, but for people who may be just naive, it is more difficult to ask for help. To come forward is a way of making yourself vulnerable ... it feels very frightening and daunting.

By talking about the links between inter-cultural work and values, this quote draws attention to the ways in which the very uncertainties of practice – that also often hold implications for forms of discrimination – are those same areas that can be actively suppressed within multiculturalism. Thus, the suppression of areas of ambiguity can actually hide and entrench forms of racism, serving simultaneously to delegitimize processes of exploration, that could uncover and challenge discriminatory practices.

To suggest that ambiguity should be recognized as a funda-mental characteristic of inter-cultural work, does not necessarily mean that practice, and particularly discriminatory practice(s), should become unaccountable. Rather, what I am suggesting is that instances of ambiguity, ambivalence and dilemma, the strategies that staff use to negotiate these areas of practice, and the emotions that go with them, should be openly interrogated and in some cases shared, as a part of the service development process. Throughout such hazardous work, the emergent nature of continually changing experiences of ethnicity can mean that any certainties of practice may exist only temporarily and then only in relation to a limited range of cases. The ambiguity of inter-cultural work should therefore be seen and used as a creative part of a necessarily unstable process of generating temporary understandings and practices, and not as a means to permanent, inflexible, solutions.

Holistic care?

In this penultimate section, I want to address some psycho-social dimensions of ethnicity that have been particularly neglected within research and models of holistic care. In many ways, attention to difference can be seen as an integral part of holistic care, that is based upon responding to 'dying patients' social, physical, psychological and spiritual needs' (Field 1989: 29). It is not surprising therefore that more recent developments in palliative care service provision have involved attention to multicultural initiatives (Hill and Penso 1995). However, despite awareness of the need to address ethnic and cultural differences in the implementation of holistic care, I found that in my research there was often an inadequate understanding amongst staff about the ways in which ethnicity, and social inequalities in particular, could affect palliative care needs (for a discussion about the more general links between inequalities and health see Dyson and Smaje, this volume).

During my research I took part in 33 in-depth interviews, with 23 service users of Asian, African and African-Caribbean descent. Although there were commonalities in the way people talked about their experiences, there were also significant differences between them that related to differences in ethnicity, culture, gender, class and migration. These differences affected how people talked about expectations of service provision, feelings of entitlement, the meaning or meaningless of terminal illness, feelings of belonging and how people died. Most significantly, I found a range of psycho-social experiences of ethnicity and culture that had direct implications for the types of support offered by palliative care services. For example, a recurrent theme in the interviews related to accounts of racism and discrimination. Nasreen, an African woman of 29, who migrated to Britain in 1984 told me 'Where I live it was by the sea . . . you don't see a black person. So when you go on the street . . . we'd see the curtains moving and they all come out and stand by their doors to look at you . . . that thing will go on forever, prejudice, racism and all that. That's for life. . . .'

Nasreen then went on to tell me about her white partner's ex-wife and family:

... they came and filled my bed with water, flooded the house ... broke all the things. Took my clothes, burnt them and left a note telling me 'if you don't leave, you'll be burnt like ashes' ... I think they would have killed me ... I had to leave ... (my) husband told me 'let's go' and I said 'no even if you took me anywhere your people would follow me ... they don't want you with a black woman'.

There are obviously many ways in which such experiences affect people, many of which are too complex or hidden to interpret fully. However, what is important is that such experiences can be neglected by the inability or unwillingness of practitioners to provide specific recognition and support for the ways in which social inequalities, such as racism can affect disease, physical, emotional and spiritual pain and caring relationships. For instance, my interview with Maxine, a Jamaican woman of 63, was interlaced with accounts of physical violence. For Maxine, her subjection to years of domestic violence was related to her cultural, rural and generational background and also to experiences of migration. Under pressure from her parents, she left Jamaica to join her husband in England during the 1960s. She told me, 'Back home, in the country they lift husband higher than God'. She wept on the plane journey to England fearing continuing violence when she joined her husband here. Once in this country, she also faced episodes of racist violence, one event when she was seven months pregnant and another so severe she thought she would lose an eye. When Maxine was admitted into the hospice for terminal care, it was noted that she would become in the words of her nurses 'anxious' and 'paranoid' during aspects of physical care. In fact, during our second interview, Maxine spontaneously described an incident of being washed by nurses where she talked about feeling frightened and objectified 'like a piece of meat'. Although it is impossible to 'prove', I feel that there were links between Maxine's experiences of physical violence and her fear and anxiety around physical contact with hospice staff. However, what is important is that such links are presently unexplored within existing models of multiculturalism and holistic care and what remains a central problem is finding ways of working, through which these links can be recognized and responded to.

Other psycho-social dimensions of ethnicity and culture that have relevance for the support offered to service users relate to feelings of identity and loss. Such emotions are a common experience for dying people of all ethnicities, who can grieve the loss of family, friends, places and things. I found that these emotions took on very specific meanings for some Asian, African and African-Caribbean people that were frequently unaddressed within holistic care. For instance, nearly all the staff interviews contained descriptions of people from these ethnic groups wanting to return to 'homelands' to die or for burial. These practices were always framed as cultural practices. For instance, when I asked one nurse about why she thought an African woman whom she had been talking about had wanted to 'return' to Africa to die, she said:

> Well I suppose that she has some sort of calling to go home. I mean by all appearances she looked sort of very modern, but I think she had some very, sort of traditional values which were quite important to her and maybe she has some sort of homing instinct or something. . . .

There are a mixture of deterministic themes in this extract which make reference to issues of culture and biology, references which were quite common in the ways some staff tried to make sense of the behaviours of different ethnic groups of service users. However, I found that in talking to service users themselves about their concepts of 'home' and also their thoughts about where they wanted to die or be buried, that these representations were also often powerful emotional and social commentaries that not only entailed negotiating dimensions of cultural identity, but also involved more generalised feelings of belonging, loss and separation. Nasreen told me that she wanted to be buried in Africa, in her family burial ground, while simply stating, 'I'd love to die in my Mum's, or in my Dad's hands'. Morris, an African-Caribbean man who lived in a high-rise, grey, inner-city, tower block, used imagery involving greenery and unbounded space, talking about his soul being able to 'fly' if he was buried in his family home in Jamaica. Ibrahim, an African, man with a young son, told me of his wish to be buried in Ghana, that:

> . . . it is my home, not in terms of religion, but . . . I want my son to . . . one day not just melt away into this society, but think of a place where he comes from and one day, or once in a while go back there, and

> when he goes there and then there's this grave stone standing there and say 'Oh there's your Dad lying down there', just to give him some kind of attachment to a place which I will cherish . . . But if he stays here, (he) just melts away into society and that's the end. . . .

While recognizing that some of these experiences involve elements of fantasy, they can nevertheless have consequences for understanding the ways in which some people negotiate feelings of loss for family and friends, for elements of their former lives or for separation from their loved ones. Most significantly, these experiences can be negated or misrepresented by subsuming their emotional significance under cultural labels. Despite the emphasis upon the need for palliative care to provide 'holistic care' that addresses individual needs, I found that this emphasis could be compromised or deflected by a preoccupation with the role of cultural prescription in the lives of people from different ethnic groups. As one member of staff told me:

> . . . the most quoted phrase which drives me up the wall . . . is, 'it's cultural'. Anything that anybody does who's not white, that is at all different in some way, 'it's cultural' and what 'it's cultural' I think means is 'we therefore do not do anything with it', because that means 'it's cultural – therefore we leave it well alone'. So that can cover anything from 'no we don't like morphine', to denying that we are dying, to the family denying that.

Within this account, the speaker places the need of some hospice staff to identify 'cultural' phenomena amongst the experiences of minority ethnic service users, with choices about professional intervention. In her interpretation, the label 'cultural' serves as both a process of 'othering' and as a means to legitimise particular 'no-go' areas for staff intervention. What is of particular interest within this example is the way in which the behaviours of white people are positioned outside of such culturalist labelling. In this way white ethnicities are not primarily 'culturalized', but are seen as being able to contain, sustain and integrate a diversity of behaviours and practices (Bonnett 1996). Hence, for some staff, the experiences of some white people can be more readily addressed individualistically under approaches of holistic care, while the experiences of minority ethnic people may be more easily culturalized away.

Conclusion

By examining different aspects of inter-cultural service provision, a central message in this chapter is that multiculturalism can often fail to respond adequately to difference and can sometimes even generate or compound existing inequalities. In relation to food, I have shown how some service initiatives can fail to recognize the changing nature of different cultural identifications, their relations to disease and how these can affect choices for service users of all ethnicities. The implications of such complex dynamics for professional practice have further suggested that multiculturalism can inhibit the productive exploration of the 'messiness' of inter-cultural work, making it difficult for staff to openly address and explore some of the more challenging aspects of their work. In giving specific attention to psycho-social experiences of difference, I have also argued that there is an inadequate understanding of the ways in which social inequalities and emotional dimensions of ethnicity and culture can affect experiences of dying and the implementation of holistic care.

However, these areas are not simply about individual practice. To work effectively and creatively with these complex issues, practitioners also need formal support and management around inter-cultural work. In this respect the recognition of ambiguity within inter-cultural service provision has much to offer. Precisely because areas of practice marked by uncertainty frequently also entail a crisis of meaning, they can serve to make explicit any gaps in organizational frameworks, while also revealing the tensions, difficulties, creativity and resources available within particular interactional sites and professional roles. Thus, a rethinking of inter-cultural practice, must also involve a move away from the securities of categorical thinking that have bedevilled attempts to respond to difference. In the tradition of holistic care there is an urgent need to develop more open, questioning and empowering forms of practice, that can resist the pressures to find simple, handy and manageable solutions to address the ever moving complexities of lived experiences.

9 Working with families from minority ethnic communities

Mel Chevannes

Introduction

In this chapter the work of community nurses with families from minority ethnic communities is examined. The work of community nurses has, until recently, paid little attention to the lived experiences of minority ethnic families. Moreover, while the work of health visitors in improving the health of families has been assessed, the role of minority ethnic families themselves in nurturing health has been neglected.

The chapter begins by outlining some current inequalities in the provision of community health services. There then follows a description of the context of community nursing for minority ethnic families. This context includes the expanded emphasis on delivery of health services through primary care groups and trusts, and the varieties of types and experiences of minority ethnic groups. In working with families within any community, it is important that nurses are aware of the changing context of household structure and family life. The chapter thus continues with an examination of recent research on the changing context of household structure and families in minority ethnic communities. The ways in which community nurses engage with families from minority ethnic communities is discussed, illustrating some of the professionally focused activities which dominate the relationship. It is argued that many of the present activities of community nurses leave little opportunity for the processes of ethnic identification and appropriate family-centred interests to claim a prominent place on the agenda of partnership between nurses and families from minority ethnic communities.

Inequalities of access to community health services

The importance of community nurses working with families from minority ethnic communities is underlined by official recognition of the health needs of minority ethnic groups (Department of Health 1990a: 26; 1991, 1993c; Johnson 1992). There has also been a growing awareness of inequitable delivery of health services to minority ethnic groups (Ahmad 1993; Smaje 1995a) and community health services in particular (Smaje 1995a; Nazroo 1997a). This is despite several authors stressing the need to provide services on an equitable basis (Blakemore 1982; Chevannes 1995), the need to promote anti-discriminatory practice (NHS Management Executive 1993); a new approach to improving health for minority ethnic groups (Department of Health 1999: 115); and the need for health professionals to be more responsive to the needs of minority ethnic communities (Gerrish *et al.* 1996).

There has been relatively little research into ethnic differences in the use of primary care services, with the exception of GP consultations. Early studies of ethnic differences in GP consultations are of limited value since they do not control for population morbidity (Balarajan *et al.* 1989; McCormick and Rosenbaum 1990). More recent surveys have employed a more comprehensive model which takes into account not only morbidity but also age, gender and socio-economic status. Benzeval and Judge (1993) in a nationally representative household survey found that after adjusting for these factors, South Asian people were more likely to consult with GPs than whites, although no significant differences in the utilization of hospital care were found. This finding was confirmed in a national survey by carried out by the Health Education Authority (Rudat 1994) and by the Policy Studies Institute survey (Nazroo 1997a). Chinese respondents at all levels of health status were less likely than others to have consulted with their GP. Smaje and Le Grand (1997) noted the under-use of GPs among Pakistani females, who showed nearly 30 per cent lower levels of utilization than their white peers.

Although there is no 'under-use' of GP consultations by most ethnic minority groups, there is some evidence to suggest that the quality of the consultations might be less than adequate.

Members of ethnic minority groups are significantly more likely than white groups to describe access to their GPs surgery as difficult (Rudat 1994). There is evidence that in general, patients from minority ethnic groups experience longer waiting times at the surgery before being seen by their GP. A study carried out for the Health Education Authority (HEA) showed that overall, ethnic minority populations were less likely than the general population to be happy with the outcome of their consultation. One in eight of the general population were unhappy, compared with one in five Caribbeans, Indians and Pakistanis and more than one in four Bangladeshis. More than three-quarters of Pakistani and Bangladeshi women expressed a preference to see a female doctor yet these preferences were not being met in a significant proportion of cases (Rudat 1994). The lack of trained interpreters in many community settings, leads to the inappropriate use of children and other family members as interpreters (Ahmad *et al.* 1989; Pharoah 1995).

There has been very little research on the use of other community health services by minority ethnic groups. The existing evidence suggests that contact with other members of the primary care team and access to a wider range of community health and social services is limited for most minority groups compared with whites. The HEA survey (Rudat 1994) shows much lower use of members of the primary care team other than GPs, especially practice nurses and district nurses. Use of health visitors and family planning clinics was broadly similar for all ethnic groups. Ethnic minority groups were less likely to have used dental services and use of chiropody services was much lower than for the UK wide sample, despite a raised incidence of diabetes in most minority ethnic groups.

The use of district nursing services is an area which gives rise to particular concern. A small number of studies which have included use of district nurses services, have highlighted some major problems for elders in particular (Norman 1985; Donaldson 1986; Pharoah 1995). A small-scale qualitative study of the up-take of district nursing services by elders in Bristol revealed a very low up-take among Asian elders in particular (Hek 1991). A similar finding emerged from a larger study of community care services for 'black' people in central Birmingham (Cameron *et al.* 1988). Blakemore (1982) notes that despite a high incidence of consultations with general practitioners, 99 per cent of Asian and 97 per cent of Caribbean older people living in Birmingham had never seen a health visitor, while over 95 per cent of both Asian and Caribbeans had never seen a district nurse (Pharoah 1995). Similar findings are also available in relation to Chinese older people (Chiu 1989), and Indian Sikh women (Boneham 1989). Lack of ethnic monitoring of community settings is a major stumbling block to developing sensitive and relevant services (Aspinall 2000).

Community social services have also been heavily criticized for ignoring the needs of minority ethnic groups, despite the policy guidance which surrounded the National Health Service and Community Care Act 1990 (Department of Health 1990b; Twigg and Atkin 1994). Ahmad and Atkin (1996: 3–5) identify three main themes underlying current inequitable provision of care in the community:

- Structural barriers in service provision, such as inability of services to support people who do not speak English or services that do not provide halal or vegetarian food choice in day care or domiciliary services.
- Overemphasis on 'cultural' practices that lead to blaming of minority ethnic groups for not making 'appropriate' use of services.
- Racist attitudes on the part of staff providing services, labelling minority ethnic clients as 'high risk', 'uncooperative' 'difficult' 'trivial complainers' or 'time wasters'.

The overall picture, then, is one of a preparedness to use the GP, but with reportedly lower levels of satisfaction. This is apparently exacerbated by lower usage of practice nurses, and district nurses, and by inequitable provision of community care services.

The context of community nursing

This section considers a number of contextual factors relating to the delivery of community health nursing care to minority ethnic communities. These factors include professional requirements; the advent of primary care trusts; and variations in the experiences of minority ethnic families.

Community nurses work outside of hospitals and nursing homes to provide healthcare services to families and individuals. They include children's nurses, district nurses, health visitors, practice nurses, learning disability nurses, mental health nurses and school nurses. The importance of community nurses working with families from minority ethnic communities is underlined by an official recognition of health needs among an ethnically diverse population and the requirement to respond to their needs by providing appropriate services (Department of Health 1990a: 26; 1991, 1993c; Johnson 1992).

Professional requirements specify that all nurses who successfully complete pre-registration courses should be able to demonstrate an 'appreciation of the influence of social, political and cultural factors in relation to health care' (Nurses, Midwives and Health Visitors (Registered Fever Nurses) Amendment Rules 1989: No. 1456, Rule 18a). The post-1995 curriculum for post-registration community nursing education (UKCC 1998) also requires them to provide services which reflect a multicultural society. Theoretically then, all community nurses should be able to meet the healthcare needs of minority ethnic communities. However, this falls short of a requirement either to challenge racism (Department of Health 1999) in service delivery or to advocate on behalf of clients experiencing racism.

The practice of nurses working with families from minority ethnic communities, as with other families, also has to be addressed in the context of the developing primary care groups and trusts (Department of Health 1997; NHS Development Unit 1998). It is intended that this will lead to family members receiving more care, treatment, and services in their homes and in the community, spending shorter times in acute hospitals, or having treatment provided on a day attendance basis to a hospital (Farrar 1999: 5). These patterns of provision are likely to lead to more health screening undertaken in general practices, combined with care provided at health centres, community hospitals, and in the home. Many of these services will be provided by different community nurses. As primary care groups achieve NHS trust status, commissioning of 'hospital' at home, and other care provided in the context of the family and the community will increase. However, this risks exacerbating exist-ing inequities in providing formal community services because of stereotyping that assumes that Asian, African and Caribbean peoples 'look after their own' (Atkin and Rollings 1996) and therefore do not require help from professional services.

The context of community nursing will also be affected by the variations *within* minority ethnic communities served. The nature of the experience of minority ethnic families is likely to depend upon many factors. For example, the particular circumstances and nature of the migration of people or their ancestors is significant. Different strata of society may have migrated, and to understand the particular needs of a local community a community nurse may need to appreciate whether the migration was composed of pro-fessionals, business middle classes, urban or rural groups, traders, students, or workers (Ahmad 1996b). Minority ethnic groups vary in kind and size in dif-ferent parts of the country (see Ahmad 1996b: 52), and this variation may be one of several contextual factors that influences the receipt of professional services. Thus the experience of Caribbeans in London, where around 60 per cent of Caribbeans in the UK live, may be very different from the 1 per cent of Caribbeans who live in East Anglia.

Community nurses need to plan care and provide services which are appropriate to, and meet health needs in line with the minority ethnic family's regime (Chevannes 1997). An under-standing of the nature of family structures and dynamics is an important part of the knowledge base of a community health nurse, necessary though not sufficient to enable her to work in an anti-discriminatory manner with families from minority ethnic communities.

Understanding family

In all ethnic groups family forms may be changing and giving way to different or new configurations, for example, lone parent households; the (re-)emergence of grandparents as key carers of children; children with parents from different ethnic groups; and two or more families living together to provide support in times of stress and adversity (Phoenix 1991; Modood *et al.* 1994; Beishon *et al.* 1998). However, Beishon *et al.* (1998: 13) caution against making generalizations that 'all the important contemporary trends are pointing in the same direction'. It is therefore important to consider the nature of minority ethnic families in contemporary Britain.

Rather than seeing a married couple with their own biological children living together in the same household unit as either 'natural' or 'the norm', the particular form relationships, families and household structures take may be thought of as a product of wider societal forces. These include the overall standard of living, social security payments, access to housing, employment opportunities, the influence of technologies such as contraception and labour-saving devices in the home, moral influences embracing attitudes to sex, contraception, abortion and socio-political influences such as the relative balance of power between men, women and children (Berthoud and Beishon 1997). The result, as Berthoud and Beishon (1997) describe, is extremely complex and liable to be easily misinterpreted. Some major factors relating to minority ethnic families and households are summarized below:

- *British-born or migrant?* Almost all minority ethnic children born to Caribbean, Indian, African Asian, Pakistani, Bangladeshi and Chinese parents (the main ethnic groupings considered in the 1997 Policy Studies Institute survey) were born in Britain.
- *First-, second- or third-generation migrants?* For the 1991–6 period, one-sixth of Pakistani and Bangladeshi, one quarter of Indian and African Asian and three-quarters of Caribbean infants had at least one British-born ethnic minority parent. Many minority ethnic under-fives visited by health visitors will therefore be third-generation migrants.
- *Cohabitation.* It is important to bear in mind the possibility, unexplored by the PSI survey, that stable partnerships, married or not, may exist without partners living together. Overall, 18 per cent of Caribbean and 11 per cent of white respondents described themselves as living as if married. Berthoud and Beishon (1997) suggest a combination of generation effect (people more willing to cohabit than in years past) and age effect (people

cohabiting when young and marrying later). This pattern did not apply to the same extent in South Asian groups, where only 2–4 per cent described themselves as cohabiting.

- *Mixed-ethnicity relationships* – 20 per cent of Caribbean, 17 per cent of Chinese, 4 per cent of Indians and African Asians and 1 per cent of Pakistanis and Bangladeshis reported having a white partner, either married or unmarried. These proportions are likely to increase over time given that the proportion tends to be higher if the minority ethnic partner was born in Britain. For Caribbeans and South Asians, two-thirds of those entering mixed ethnic partnerships were men, although for Chinese two-thirds were women. For children whose mother and father lived with them, 39 per cent of Caribbean, 15 per cent of Chinese, 3 per cent of Indian/African-Asian and 1 per cent of Pakistani/Bangladeshi children had one white parent.

- *Separation, divorce and widowhood.* Six per cent of Pakistanis and Bangladeshis were together but living apart from partners for work reasons compared to 1–2 per cent in other groups; 18 per cent of Caribbean, 9 per cent of white and 4 per cent of Asians had separated without remarrying. Analysis of differences in rates of separation by age group suggests that Caribbean marriages have been ending at higher rates for a number of years and that white separations are beginning to follow this rising trend.

- *Formal marriage.* Overall, 58 per cent of whites, 73 per cent of South Asians and 39 per cent of Caribbeans under 60 are formally married. Nevertheless formal marriage was the most common single outcome for Caribbeans as it was for whites and Asians.

- *Children.* South Asian groups are more likely than other ethnic groups to have children and to have greater number of children against an historical trend of later and fewer children. This will have consequences not only for family structure but also for their standard of living. Couples from all minority ethnic groups, including Caribbeans, were more likely than whites to have children.

- *Lone parents.* The conventional order of analysis asking first about marriage and then about children is revealed to be inappropriate for Caribbean women, and increasingly for white women; 47 per cent of 'never-married' Caribbean women and 16 per cent of equivalent white women had children.

- *Size of family.* Chinese families have slightly fewer children on average than whites. Caribbean and African Asian family sizes are the same as whites, Indian families having slightly more children on average. However, the pattern of starting families early and continuing to have children into their forties that is characteristic of Pakistani and Bangladeshi women is behind the figures of 33 per cent Pakistani and 42 per cent Bangladeshi families who have four or more children. Berthoud and Beishon (1997) argue that British social policy has lost sight of the issue of the large family. The difficulties experienced by Pakistani and Bangladeshi people in the labour market, together with poor housing bring about particular challenges for these families, many of whom live in considerable poverty.
- *Households.* Table 9.1 suggests that different social circumstances and age structures of ethnic groups lead to different patterns of household composition.
- *Contacts with kin.* It is important that nurses do not make assumptions about likely or possible sources of social support. Berthoud and Beishon (1997) remind us that Caribbeans, Pakistanis and Bangladeshis in particular may have parents abroad, lack social support because of family separation across countries, and have reduced income owing to obligations to remit monies to help relatives abroad. They also point out that South Asian and Caribbean families are more likely to have adult offspring still living in the parental home. They note the high degree of contact, by telephone and letter, of various minority ethnic groups, and the stronger horizontal ties in minority groups (e.g. to aunts and uncles) as well as vertical ones (to parents and children).
- *Caring.* Berthoud and Beishon (1997) note that Caribbeans are less likely to be caring for older parents. Rates for whites and South Asians are similar (once the effect of parents separated abroad is taken into account) though whites tend to be providing the support from a

Table 9.1 Household structure in percentages by 1991 classification of ethnic group.

	White	Caribbean	Indian/ African- Asian	Pakistani/ Bangladeshi	Chinese
One or two adults, either 60+	30	14	7	3	7
One adult less than 60	11	14	4	3	13
Two adults both less than 60	18	14	9	6	10
One adult with children	5	17	3	3	3
Two adults, 1–2 children	15	19	26	14	20
Two adults, 3 or 3+ children	4	5	9	21	8
Three+ adults, with/without children	17	18	42	49	40

Source: Adapted from Berthoud and Beishon (1997: 46).

separate household rather than from within the same household.

Any assumption about the existence of a single family pattern for minority ethnic groups denies important differences brought about by geographical change, urbanization, processes of ethnic identification and racism, and between first-, second- and third-generation families from the New Commonwealth living in the UK (Modood *et al.* 1994). An understanding of diversity is important contextual information since an awareness of family and household forms should inform the kinds of interventions taken by community nurses.

While it is necessary to learn from families about, for example, how they care and support themselves within the diversity of households to be found among minority ethnic families (Beishon *et al.* 1998: 16, 37–8), it is vital not to overemphasize the differences between ethnic minority and ethnic majority families. It is also important for nurses to be sensitive to divisions within families which can affect access to health resources. For example, there are dangers in assuming that men, women and children, have equal access to resources and life chances in households (Townsend 1979; Townsend *et al.* 1988; Graham 1992). It is women in black Caribbean and South Asian households, as well as white, who most often take the major responsibility for the care of children, family shopping, meals, and housekeeping (Afshar 1989; Chevannes 1989; Phoenix 1991; Beishon *et al.* 1998). However, women are less likely to have access to car use (Townsend *et al.* 1988). This relative lack of car use points to a greater unevenness between men and women in resources for family health, because shopping and taking the children to general practitioners, or health visitors during the day, are frequently undertaken by women (Townsend *et al.* 1988; Graham 1992).

Overall the patterns of kinship, households and social support are complex, varied and changing. It is important not to overemphasize the differences between ethnic groups, and not to see variations in family forms as 'naturally' a consequence of ethnicity, but as an outcome of complex social, economic and cultural circumstances.

Community and minority ethnic groups

It has been noted above that inequitable provision of professional community health services may reflect stereotypes that assume that minority ethnic groups provide greater levels of informal care in the community (Atkin and Rollings 1996). Once again, contextual social factors may produce differences that could be misread as the effects of ethnicity.

Modood *et al.* (1994) and Beishon *et al.* (1998) note that three of the main features that separate minority ethnic families from others relate to the effects of geographical change, urbanization, and racism on family life. In particular, the family as a 'resource' to protect family members against racism and discrimination (Beishon *et al.* 1998) clearly has more resonance with minority ethnic families than with ethnic majority families because of the shared experience of racism and discrimination.

In cases where minority ethnic communities have migrated from small scale rural living to urban life (Modood *et al.* 1994) there may be particular challenges for community nurses to address in supporting such groups. Currer (1986) notes how for Pathan women, migrated from rural Pakistan, the urban spaces of Bradford precluded the gender-specific support networks for which specific space within village life had existed. Moreover, kinship networks often carry with them specific family and community obligations. Ahmad (1996b), for example, discusses the *biarderi* – a Punjabi term for a kinship based group that places expectations upon its members that they will offer mutual moral, financial, and social help.

Technological developments such as rapid transport, telephone and other electronic means of communication have expanded kinship relations beyond traditional geographical boundaries. Berthoud and Beishon (1997) note that contact between kin involves not only personal contact but letters and phone calls between areas or even between countries. It is also important to note the example of working-class Caribbean women in Hackney for whom church was an important source of social support (Gabe and Thorogood 1986), a reminder that quality social support need not only be family or kin-based. The church forms a common place of collective activity for many first- and second-generation Caribbean people, and for others, it is voluntary organizations or youth groups (Reeves 1989: 30–37). The coming together of a group of women to challenge racism and racial discrimination in a locality is an example of a 'community' based on common interests (Cohen 1985). The Southall Black Sisters is an example of a 'community' based on common interests (Cohen 1985). This group of women came together initially to combat racism faced by Asians and Caribbeans in Southall and later extended their activities to wider social and political issues.

In summary, this section suggests that family support may have different levels of importance for those facing racism; that kinship networks take many forms, and both offer support and demand obligations; and that quality social support may derive from non-kin sources such as churches or political groups.

Professionals and health surveillance

The author's experiences of health visitor supervision suggests that, typically, families' experiences and health needs are interpreted by community nurses within their own professional framework. For example, a white English-speaking health visitor visits an Indian family at their home to monitor the physical and social development of a 12-months-old child. The mother who is engaged in preparing pokoras, welcomes the unexpected health visitor into the home by using English words in a limited way. Following friendly and polite exchanges between the mother and the health visitor, the mother is asked in English about a number of growth and development milestones expected of a 12-months-old child. The mother tries really hard to speak in English as she asks the health visitor for more information in an attempt to understand the questions. After some time, in which the health visitor questions the mother using gestures, and emphasizing words loudly, the exchange stops. The health visitor then observes the child who walks around the room and utters short words she (health visitor) does not understand. The health visitor says goodbye and departs from the family home to record her assessment of the visit, primarily in terms of child developmental achievements and shortcomings.

In this situation, the service provided by the health visitor could have been greatly improved with the involvement of either a bilingual health worker or by an interpreter trained to understand and translate information about children's development, and competent in the language spoken by the mother. It has been noted elsewhere (Pharoah 1995) that some health visitors, district nurses, and general practitioners avoid minority ethnic families where they are required to spend more time to understand what the family says. The professionals' lack of knowledge about the processes by which the family are developing their culture, and their perceived behaviour of these families also reduce the level of contact. This example of the health visitor's work illustrates three issues worthy of further comment – time to communicate, needs being unmet, and child development surveillance measures.

The first issue highlighted by the health visitor example discussed above is the time required to communicate where the two main speakers are competent in a different language. The inability of the English-speaking health visitor to converse with the mother who is competent in Punjabi impedes the quality of the discussion about the child's development. It will impede the health visitor in explaining the purpose of the visit, and the reasons for the questions asked. Similarly, the mother will experience difficulty in describing how she sees her child's development, the child's use of Punjabi words, the Indian meals she eats, and the support provided by other family members. In this situation, more time is required by the health visitor to listen, hear, understand, and respond to the mother. The exchange will require an enormous investment of time both for the health visitor and the mother and yet still vital information will be missed. The employment of properly trained interpreters, or health visitors who are also competent to converse in the language used by mothers from minority ethnic backgrounds, is vital to the integrity of the exchange.

The second issue is a lack of proper developmental assessment of the 12-months-old child by the health visitor. While there may be a close approximation between the child's locomotor skills, exemplified by walking and the health visitor's observation, assessment of the child's development in interactive social skills, manipulative skills, ability to feed herself, speech and language may not be carried out effectively or at all. This failure leaves the child and her mother without the benefit of knowing the child's development in the fields outlined. An early identification of developmental delay in any field of a child's growth is suggested to be a major benefit of health surveillance to the child and the family (Court 1976). The child in the above example may miss out on early intervention in the event of delayed development because the health visitor was unable to undertake her assessment. Also important is a failure on the part of the health visitor to be accountable to her employer for a service which should be provided to the child and the family.

The third issue concerns the nature of the surveillance measures used by health visitors to assess the development of all children at prescribed chronological ages. The surveillance of young children's development is part of a portfolio of milestones expected to be reached by children at set ages aged from birth up to five years. The schedule of milestones is, in the main, devised on the achievement of white children in the British (see Griffiths 1960) or American population (see Denver scale, Frankenburg and Dodds 1967). Some changes have been made to the surveillance measures (see Moreton and MacFarlane 1991; Hall DM 1996) to take account of the development of children from black and other minority ethnic communities. If surveillance measures are to be used, it is important that the expected standards of all children's development are based on a representative sample of children from all ethnic groups. Otherwise this leaves community health nurses vulnerable: are they discriminating if they apply the same parameters or are they discriminating if they apply different parameters?

Recent health reforms (Department of Health 1999), including primary care trusts (Farrar 1999), place an increasing emphasis on adults and children contributing to their own health assessment. An example from the author's professional practice suggests that this health policy has not been incorporated into the work of community nursing. In a Moslem family, a child who is recovering from a bout of asthma and is away from school expresses a wish to attend classes at the local mosque where the environment is relaxed, friendly, and supportive. The child's wish for this activity as part of his treatment plan, and supported by his parents, conflicts with the health visitor's advice which stresses that he should stay at home as he is not yet fit to return to school.

In this situation, the model of community participation advocated by the World Health Organization (1993) may provide, for health visitors, a way of working to incorporate the families' views. The model of community participation emphasizes the benefits to families, the wider community, and health professionals from working together. Extra time for community nurses to undertake this work, particularly where there are difficulties in the use of a common language, must be built into their workload. Furthermore, a recognition of the unequal power between community nurses and families, in particular children, points to a need to develop partnership working as a goal in community nursing. Developing such partnerships requires in turn the support of managers and employers as a first step towards realising less professionally dominated approaches.

Partnership between minority ethnic families and community nurses requires a willingness on the part of community nurses to be less negative about these families (Pharoah 1995), and to develop a knowledge about anti-discrimination legislation (for example, Sex Discrimination Act 1975; Race Relations Act 1976; the Disability Discrimination Act 1996; Race Relations Amendment Bill 2000). The model of community participation between community nurses and families suggested by the World Health Organization (1993) can be incorporated into three-yearly agreements about standards of care. Three-yearly agreements are intended to specify standards of care (Department of Health 1997) between commissioners and providers of health services, such as community trusts or primary care groups/trusts. These agreements could include, for example, anti-discriminatory standards of care for all families (Commission for Racial Equality 1992), including those from minority ethnic communities, and the use of appropriate surveillance tools for measuring the development of children.

New ways of working

In keeping with the principle of respecting individual privacy, dignity, religious, and cultural beliefs (UKCC 1998; NHS Executive 1995), community nurses need to work in partnership, adopt non-discriminatory measures, and develop ways of working with minority ethnic families that do not stereotype them. There is a wealth of information (see NHS Executive 1992; Health Education Authority 1994; Pharoah 1995; Jamdagni 1996) *but this information needs to be critically evaluated by community nurses* before it can be used in their work with families from minority ethnic communities.

For example, nurses may have access to 'checklists' of what health professionals should know about minority ethnic communities (see for example, Henley 1983; Karmi 1996; Smith and Pankhania 1996). Karmi (1996) argues that such checklists provide accessible information about the cultures and norms of minority ethnic groups, which health professionals can assimilate rapidly. However, Gunaratnam (1993) stresses that such guides are only a starting point to develop an awareness among professionals concerning in what domains of experience (food, religion, washing, dress) there may be relevant variation in client preferences. Such information therefore only represents the raw material from which to construct reflexive nursing practice and *not* the achievement of such practice.

A guide, on is own, is no substitute for a proper understanding of the basis of practices and the experience of working with particular minority ethnic families (Department of Health 1998c). There is a need to incorporate the experiences of individual family members and the family as a whole as they strive to look after themselves. For example, a male teenager from an Indian Sikh family living in Southall may fear racist behaviour and possibly physical violence when he ventures from the family home, leading him to absenting himself from school, refusing food excessively, and creating undue tension among the parents (Young 1999).

Nurses may also make use of information that describes specific local initiatives and projects which have been designed to improve the access of minority ethnic users to a range of services (Health Education Authority 1994; Department of Health 1996). The NHS Confederation has published a composite list of projects which have been funded by the NHS ethnic health unit. Many of these explore in detail the problems experienced by minority ethnic users of primary care and issues faced by primary healthcare teams in delivering culturally appropriate services (NHS Confederation 1998).

Community nurses may also have access to policy materials that advocate the need to improve health services and to reduce inequalities in health (Acheson 1998). Central to both aims is the importance of hearing the views and experiences of individuals from their respective minority ethnic communities (NHS Executive 1992; Kapasi 1995). Kapasi's (1995) work in Sandwell with black older people from Indian and Caribbean backgrounds who had suffered a stroke and were hospitalised provides useful information for community nurses with responsibility for such patients when they return to their home. For example, older Indians needed individuals who were bilingual to advocate for them (Kapasi 1995: 21). Also highlighted was the need for staff to be knowledgeable about services available for stroke sufferers, and an understanding of and respect for the social processes by which the diverse peoples of Indian and Caribbean descent were engaged in developing their lifestyles, culture, and religion (Kapasi 1995: 17, 23).

These examples of initiatives that insufficiently involve minority ethnic communities and individuals reminds us that families should be seen as active participants in their own health care, having the ability to understand their health experiences, and to identify their health concerns (Hartrick 1994). In this sense, work-based learning could be used as part of a portfolio of continuing professional development of community nurses.

Work-based learning could be developed through the full involvement of the minority ethnic families concerned. Work-based learning is a dynamic and structured process which requires community nurses to develop different ways of working. These different ways include

- shifting from using an imposed professional style with families;
- avoiding stereotyping individuals from any ethnic group;
- understanding how a disease like diabetes, outside of drug therapy, can be managed within the culture of the family; and
- having greater knowledge about the use of foods used by family members to create an emergent culture.

In this context, work-based learning affords an opportunity to community nurses to become co-learners with families about health management in a culturally safe way. In working with families with diabetes, for example, community nurses are expected to be able to inform individuals about the physiology, and the technical treatment of the disease. Equally important, however, is the need to go beyond the physiological and technical knowledge of diabetes, to those practices and behaviours which families believe to be conducive to their health maintenance, and integral to their processes of ethnic identification. For example, a Black Caribbean mother may describe a range of Caribbean foods, for example, ginger cake with very little molasses, rice and peas without adding creamed coconut, small quantities of hard and soft yams, and unsweetened carrot juice she prepares and eats as part of her diet to help manage the diabetes. Here the mother provides the community nurse responsible for the management of her diabetes with an opportunity to learn about the contextual use of appropriate foods to create a dietary practice that is both clinically and culturally safe. As Gunaratnam (Chapter 8, this volume) argues, food is one resource used in many ways, including in the management of illness, and is therefore best thought of as a resource to actively *create* culture rather than being a reflection of culture.

Community nurses may also develop their knowledge and understanding of weaning by learning which foods some Black Caribbean women may use to assist their children to wean from an all milk diet to solid food. They may also develop a more dynamic understanding of religion in context by appreciating the purpose of an open section of the bible in a baby's cot to display selected psalms (Chevannes 1989). This learning may often be from families but community nurses are themselves from diverse ethnic backgrounds and have much to learn from one another. These practices which are not always understood and used by nurses in the context of their work with families from minority ethnic communities may, nevertheless, be critical to the family members' compliance with associated health advice. Nurses, who may be steeped in traditional and Eurocentric ways of working, may fail to understand, for example, the lack of effectiveness of a drug therapy on a Black Caribbean woman's hypertension who, unbeknown to the nurse, resorts to home cures, such as pureed bitter aloe (or more popularly known as sickle bible), and abandons the prescribed medication believing that a daily portion of bitter aloe is more effective.

From a sample of women who migrated from Jamaica to England, Chevannes (1989) found that the use of a 'triple insurance policy' played an important part in the care of their children's illnesses. A combination of home cures, beliefs derived from religious and ancestral sources, and professional treatment were invoked for different kinds of illnesses, ailments, and health protection generally, although not in any particular order of priority. An understanding of how these women, in the context of their families, think about and deal with their children's illnesses is essential for safe and effective ways of working.

In moving towards less professionally dominated and non-stereotypical ways of working, community nurses may create a positive framework by giving more attention to the strengths in families, learning about how they deal with constraints and difficulties in living, their experiences of managing discrimination of family members, and their responses to inappropriate or inaccessible health services. A more positive framework, underpinned by the value of learning to work with minority ethnic families, can promote the confidence of minority ethnic clients in their capacity to organize, and manage their lives in ways which are different, culturally safe, and health enhancing. An understanding of the interplay of factors from the families' points of view, for example, age of family members, parents' countries of origin, differences between the generations, experiences of health services, safety of neighbourhood, and the experience of discrimination, may assist community nurses to develop more open and non-stereotypical approaches in their work.

Conclusion

This chapter has focused on several issues which affect the work of community nurses with families from minority ethnic communities. The chapter has described inequalities of access to community health services and the context in which community nurses work. It has also described complex and changing patterns of kinship, households and social support in minority ethnic groups. The evidence indicates that minority ethnic families have experiences which are shaped by racism and on this basis differ from families who do not share such experiences. This has implications for the way community nurses work with these families in their homes, and in other primary care settings. The development of primary care trusts could challenge any work by community nurses that ignores family diversity and fails to tackle racism.

An understanding of anti-discriminatory measures and a commitment to work in partnership with minority ethnic families are suggested as positive moves away from professionally dominated ways of working. It is suggested that community nurses could use existing resources to assist them to develop less professionally dominated and non-stereotypical ways of working with families. However, the use of such resources should be within the context of an understanding of the diversity of families' experiences and behaviour. Working with families from minority ethnic communities is a critical issue as we enter the new millennium. Ethnic minority family members will expect, like other citizens, to be treated respectfully and competently by nurses. Nursing, therefore, has a responsibility to ensure that the education process equips nurses with a thorough understanding of the healthcare system, models of care, systems of diagnoses and theories of healing which take fully into account the healthcare needs of a multiethnic population. The health status of individuals from minority ethnic communities and their health improvement should be recognized as an important indication and measure of the success of the modern health services and society as a whole.

PART III

Nurses from minority ethnic groups

---

10 Ethnicity and nursing careers

Lorraine Culley and Vina Mayor

Introduction

Social scientists have played a major role in debating the economic and social position of racialized minorities in Britain since the 1950s. Extensive evidence has been gathered of ethnic disadvantage in the labour market and of discriminatory practices in employment and all major social institutions, including the education system, the welfare system and the criminal justice system (Mason 1995; Fenton 1999). This chapter discusses the experiences of nurses from minority ethnic groups in the NHS. It begins by looking briefly at the historical contribution of workers who migrated to the UK in the postwar period and goes on to examine the contemporary evidence concerning the work experiences of today's ethnic minority nurses. The chapter also discusses equal opportunities initiatives and issues relating to education and training.

Occupational position of minority ethnic groups

Patterns of global migration have been shaped by both economic and political inequalities. In the case of Britain, the particular circumstances of colonialism have determined specific features of immigration and the response to migrants (Mason 1995). There has been a presence of people of Caribbean, South Asian and African origin in Britain for centuries but it was in the post Second World War period that larger scale migration to Britain occurred, largely in response to labour shortages in key sectors of the economy (Fryer 1984). The employment of migrant labour was seen by employers and government as

a way of filling the jobs which indigenous workers were unwilling to do in the postwar economic boom. These migrant
workers entered the lower levels of the labour market
in unskilled and low paid jobs, often with unsocial hours and
poor working conditions (Mason 1995). Many migrants with
skilled or professional jobs in their country of origin nevertheless found themselves channelled by employers, white employees and their trade unions into low status jobs (Phizacklea
and Miles 1992).

Successive research studies from the 1960s onwards revealed
that many minority ethnic workers continued to be clustered in
particular industries and occupations, were over-represented in
semi-skilled and unskilled jobs and experienced higher rates of
unemployment than their white counterparts (Brown 1984).
Current research, however, presents a more complex picture,
with considerable diversity and divergence between the socio-
economic status of different minority ethnic groups. The Fourth
National Survey of Ethnic Minorities undertaken by the Policy
Studies Institute (PSI) revealed continued and persistent disadvantage for some groups, coupled with significant progress for
others (Modood *et al.* 1997). Broadly, these and other findings
demonstrate that Pakistanis and Bangladeshis are consistently at
a disadvantage with respect to white people and occupy a position of serious disadvantage on wide range of indicators including those relating to employment. People of Caribbean origin
and Indian origin are often found to experience disadvantage,
although it is usually less serious. Chinese people and African
Asians 'have reached a position of broad parity with the white
population – behind on some indicators perhaps, but ahead on
others' (Modood *et al.* 1997: 342).

Despite the fact that the National Health Service (NHS) is
the largest employer in Western Europe and a major employer
of minority ethnic workers, there has been relatively little
research on the work patterns of these workers until quite
recently. This relative invisibility of ethnicity in analyses of
NHS occupational groups, is mirrored in sociological debates
about the professions more generally. There is a notable absence
of a racial or ethnic dimension to the dominant sociological
debates on the professions and professionalism in British
sociology. Difficulties experienced by overseas doctors were

highlighted in a study nearly twenty years ago (Smith 1980) and there has been an ongoing debate in the medical press on discrimination in medicine (Commission for Racial Equality 1983; McKenzie 1995; Godlee 1996; Esmail and Everington 1993). It was not until 1995 that the first national survey of minority ethnic nurses was published (Beishon *et al.* 1995) and the research evidence on other workers such as ancillary and catering staff is very scant.

Historical background – 'overseas' nurses in the NHS

In 1998 Britain celebrated the fiftieth anniversary of two historical events of considerable significance to healthcare in the UK – 1948 was the year in which the postwar Labour Government created the new National Health Service and it was also the year in which the passenger ship *Empire Windrush* arrived in London carrying several hundred migrants from the Caribbean. This signalled the start of a pattern of immigration that has provided many workers for the NHS and other public services (Phillips and Phillips 1998).

At its inception the NHS was suffering from a severe shortage of workers and without the contribution of what were then termed 'overseas' nurses and doctors, it is difficult to see how the healthcare system could have prospered. Large numbers of migrants were also recruited into ancillary work such as domestic, catering, cleaning and maintenance jobs. An assessment of the numbers joining the NHS is difficult, because of the lack of ethnic monitoring, but one study estimated that by 1971 there were over 15,000 'overseas' nurses in the NHS (around 9 per cent of nurses), with 40 per cent described as West Indian, 29 per cent Asian and 27 per cent African (Akinsanya 1988).

Recruitment from overseas declined in the 1970s following legislation restricting immigration generally and by the mid-1980s overseas recruitment had virtually ceased. More recently this has increased again as a response to serious labour shortages (Carlisle 1996). Today, the term 'minority ethnic nurses' tends to imply not only those who have migrated to the UK but those who have been born and/or largely brought up in this country who describe their ethnic origin as other than 'white'.

As noted elsewhere in this volume, this presents particular difficulties for those minority ethnic groups who may suffer from discrimination and disadvantage but who are generally subsumed under the 'white' category – most notably in this case a significant number of nurses of Irish origin. There is very little research concerning this group of nurses and the findings on their experience of discrimination are contradictory (Snell 1997).

An early study of migrant nurses identified an under-representation of overseas nurses in senior grades and found that they were more likely to be in the less popular and less prestigious specialities such as geriatric and psychiatric nursing (Thomas and Morton-Williams 1972). There is also evidence that many who came to Britain to train as nurses were channelled into State Enrolled Nurse (SEN) training rather than the more prestigous State Registered Nurse (SRN) courses. Many others found themselves working as nursing auxiliaries (Baxter 1988; Ellis 1990). Qualitative accounts of what life was like for these nurses is very fragmentary, yet suggests that many nurses suffered extensively from racist practices of many kinds – both personal and institutional (see Chapter 11, this volume). There was little or no legal redress against most forms of direct discrimination until the Race Relations Act of 1965. Legislative protection was extended to cover employment issues in 1968 and it was not until 1976 that the Race Relations Act provided more effective protection against racial discrimination in employment.

Small scale qualitative studies carried out in the 1980s create a rather bleak picture of extensive discrimination reported by ethnic minority nurses (Baxter 1988; Lee-Cunin 1989). There was anecdotal evidence of a concentration in the lower grades and in less popular and less prestigious nursing specialties such as geriatrics and mental health; an under-representation in teaching hospitals and suggestions of discrimination in recruitment, promotion, access to training opportunities and career development generally. In 1986, the Department of Health and the King's Fund established an Equal Opportunities Task Force, which was in existence until 1990. This group highlighted a significant under-representation of minority ethnic staff in senior management positions generally in the NHS and produced the special report *Racial Equality: The Nursing Profession* (Ellis 1990). This concluded that there was evidence becoming available to support the anecdotal accounts of inequality. 'Racial inequality in the nursing profession is wide ranging and deep seated. It has been entrenched for a long time and will be difficult to remedy' (Ellis 1990: 38).

The ethnic composition of nursing in the NHS

It is only very recently that ethnic monitoring has been under-taken in the NHS and even now there is evidence that its implementation is still not universal (MSF 1997). The English National Board for Nursing, Midwifery and Health Visiting (ENB) data on the ethnic background of applicants to nurse training is incomplete and the United Kingdom Central Council for Nursing, Midwifery and Health Visiting (UKCC) has only recently begun to record the ethnic background of qualified practitioners. It is, therefore, difficult to give accurate figures for the numbers of minority ethnic personnel employed at the present time. One estimate, from the Labour Force Survey 1988–90 concludes that about 5,000 male and 3,500 female minority ethnic nurses were employed – about 8 per cent of all nursing and midwifery staff (Beishon *et al.* 1995). The largest minority ethnic group represented was the 'West Indian' group, with very few nurses from the Bangladeshi or Pakistani communities.

Beishon *et al.* (1995) also identified around 8 per cent of respondents in their national survey of over 14,000 nurses as members of minority ethnic groups. However, the overall figures conceal differences between census categories. While the black groups (Black Other, Black African and Black Caribbean) were numerically over-represented, the Asian category (Bangladeshi, Indian and Pakistani groups) were under-represented compared with the proportion of these groups in the population overall (Beishon *et al.* 1995).

It would be incorrect to assume from this data, however, that recruitment from minority ethnic groups is buoyant. Analysis of Department of Health statistics by the trade union MSF (MSF 1997) has shown a sharp drop in recruitment. This study suggested that less than 0.8 per cent of the under 25 year-olds in employment as nurses, midwives or health visitors were identified as 'black' and 1 per cent as 'Asian', although it did acknowledge large gaps in the data which may make these estimates unreliable. The largest proportion of minority ethnic nurses were in the 55–64 age group (many of these are likely to have been born outside the UK) and consequently close to retirement. At a time, therefore, when the government is concerned to increase recruitment of minority ethnic staff, this evidence suggests that fewer young people from minority ethnic groups are choosing nursing as a career.

As Iganski *et al.* (1998) have argued, there are two reasons why governments are concerned to increase minority ethnic recruitment to nursing and midwifery. First, there are assumed implications for the quality of healthcare provision to diverse communities if minority ethnic staff share the cultural and linguistic characteristics of the communities they serve. Second, minority ethnic young people are seen as an important potential source of labour in times of recruitment and retention difficulties in the profession generally. As such, therefore, if some groups were under-represented in the nursing workforce, this would represent a threat to the operational effectiveness of the NHS. These arguments will be examined in more detail later. For the moment the chapter will consider recent research evidence on the recruitment and selection of students into nurse education.

Recruitment to nurse education

Several authors have suggested that members of minority ethnic groups are being deterred from applying to the nursing profession because of the discrimination and harassment experienced by their parents' generation (Baxter 1988; Lee-Cunin 1989). However, the data on which to base such an argument have been limited. A recent analysis of the national pattern of applications from members of minority ethnic groups to pre-registration nursing and midwifery training shows a complex pattern of numerical under- and in some cases, over-representation (Iganski *et al.* 1998). This comprehensive study found that 9 per cent of applicants classified themselves into one of the black Census groups (Black Caribbean, Black African, Black Other), which represents an over-representation compared with the proportion in the population as a whole. A considerable gender difference was found, however, with 18 per cent of male applicants classifying themselves as black compared with 8 per cent of female applicants. Black Africans were strongly represented in both groups and largely accounted for the bulk of the over-representation.

In contrast, the Asian groups were numerically under-represented, with the exception of Indian males. Significant proportions of 'non-white' applicants were overseas applicants. When these applicants were excluded from the calculations, the Asian groups were still under-represented and the over-representation of the black groups was reduced, although remained overall. When calculated against those age cohorts of the population from which applicants are normally drawn, over-representation of some black groups disappears, although those identified as Black African remain over-represented.

The evidence on applications to nurse training then, shows a complex pattern across minority ethnic groups. The study also examined the *success rates* of applicants from each ethnic group and found significant differences in application outcomes between minority ethnic groups and the white group, with white applicants consistently more likely to have commenced education or be holding an offer than minority ethnic applicants. A much higher proportion of most minority ethnic groups than white groups are rejected before interview.

> These differences cannot be explained by qualification level, special-ism chosen, visa requirements, age or a combination of these. This suggests that factors in the selection process have the effect, inten-tionally or otherwise, of discriminating against some applicants on the basis of their ethnic group. (Iganski *et al.* 1998: 94)

It appears therefore, that discrimination on the grounds of ethnicity is occurring in selection for nurse training. Gerrish *et al.* (1996) also concluded that minority ethnic applicants in their study were less likely to secure a place in nurse training than white applicants. They argued that this might be partly explained by a reluctance on the part of colleges to offer places to overseas applicants because it was thought unlikely that they would obtain a work permit upon completion. Links between local workforce planning and local recruitment and subsequent retention of workers also raise concerns about the value of recruiting from overseas.

The research concludes that the predictions about the demise of the 'black nurse' (Baxter 1988) may have been premature. The apparent differences between the number of applicants from black groups and from Asian groups, seems to support the hypothesis that processes operating within some Asian communities may deter young people from these communities from pursing a career in nursing. While there are undoubtedly problems with the way in which this view is often simplistically and uncritically proposed as a 'problem' of Asian culture (Ward 1993), it is nevertheless the case that there appears to be a low level of interest in nursing as a career within some Asian communities and further research is needed into why this might be and what can be done to address it.

Ethnicity and professional education

The literature on the experiences of minority ethnic nursing students is very patchy. Day (1994) has suggested that minority ethnic students are less likely to complete professional courses. Participants in the study of nurse education undertaken by Gerrish *et al.* (1996) acknowledged the existence of racism in both the college and practice settings. Tutors reported that they felt ill equipped to challenge racist sentiments expressed in classroom settings. This 'brings into question their ability to support minority ethnic students who may be subject to racial prejudice and leaves the minority ethnic student in a particularly vulnerable and unsupported position' (Gerrish *et al.* 1996: 140). Racism in the practice setting is also a problem facing minority ethnic students, many of whom may be reluctant to complain precisely because of their student status. It may also be difficult for victims to complain to people who are of the same ethnic background as the perpetrator.

The study by Gerrish *et al.* also highlights the difficult position that minority ethnic students and staff occupy within educational institutions and the health service. The study found that there was a tendency for such students to be regarded as experts on all matters relating to ethnicity and to be seen as a resource for fellow students and for staff. 'This places a considerable and unreasonable burden on minority ethnic students and detracts from the need for such students themselves to develop the skills to work in a multi-ethnic population' (1996: 141). It also runs the risk of these individuals being seen as knowledgeable *only* on matters of ethnicity. There was little evidence in this study that educational institutions understood the potentially vulnerable position of minority ethnic students or provided specific counselling or pastoral support for students who might be exposed to racism in the placement setting.

Racism and nursing careers

It is not only at the point of recruitment and training that people from minority ethnic groups may suffer institutional and individual racism. The study carried out by the Policy Studies Institute clearly indicates the need for employers to address a range of inequalities and discrimination facing minority ethnic nursing staff (Beishon *et al.* 1995). In 1994 the Department of Health commissioned the PSI to conduct a large scale research project into the experiences of nursing and midwifery staff in the NHS. This consisted of an in-depth qualitative case study of six nurse employers, reflecting the geographical distribution of the ethnic minority population and the geographical spread of the ethnic minority nursing workforce in England, together with a nationally representative survey of nursing and midwifery staff (including auxiliaries and health visitors). The case studies were designed to examine equal opportunities policies relating to recruitment, training, appraisal and flexible working and the ways in which these impact on the experiences of staff from minority ethnic groups. The extent of racial harassment in the workplace was also a key issue examined in the case studies. The postal survey sought to provide detailed information on the current distribution of ethnic minority nursing staff across grades and specialties and possible reasons for this pattern. Although a very valuable study, it is important to make the point that the study did not include the top nursing grades for the acute sector (H and above) and did include nursing auxiliaries as well as professionally qualified staff.

The study showed several ways in which nursing staff from minority ethnic groups were disadvantaged. The results of the postal survey (14,330 respondents) revealed differences in employment characteristics and career paths of white and minority ethnic nurses. Ethnic minority nursing staff were older than white nursing staff, had fewer general educational qualifications and were more likely to be working in specialties such as mental illness and learning disabilities. The ethnic minority staff appeared to be relatively well represented in the higher grades of nursing. However, a more detailed analysis which looked at predictors of nursing level showed that although there were no indications of minorities being at a disadvantage in access to middle-ranking posts up to E grade, those in the Black categories in particular were at a significant disadvantage in access to grade F and above. Asians may also have been slower to reach these senior grades. Approximately one quarter of staff believed that they had been denied opportunities for training because of their ethnicity and the same proportion thought that they had been discriminated against in recruitment or promotion.

One of the most striking findings of this study concerned the widespread racial harassment of ethnic minority staff by patients and colleagues. This issue was included in both the postal survey and the case study interviews. In the postal survey, more than one third of nurses reported that they had suffered racial harassment by work colleagues, and more than two thirds reported being racially harassed by patients and families. Interviews with staff in the six case study areas revealed examples of harassment in all areas and across all specialties, although the extent of this varied between case study employers. In one area, several minority ethnic nurses said that they had been subjected to racial harassment from colleagues and that such racism was a regular feature of their working lives. This often took the form of unpleasantness – the day-to-day feeling that they were not liked. In one community setting, it took the form of white staff stereotyping minority ethnic groups and being openly disparaging about issues relating to ethnicity in the presence of minority ethnic staff.

Harassment by patients and their families also varied in scale and nature across the different employers and specialties within each employer. This harassment took two main forms. First, minority ethnic nurses were subjected to clear racist verbal abuse by patients and experienced situations where patients refused to be treated by them. Second, there was a more subtle form of harassment, where white patients did not explicitly mention ethnicity but clearly treated minority ethnic nurses in a relatively unfavourable way compared to white nurses. Several white nurses reported witnessing the racial harassment of minority ethnic staff.

The study found that most incidents of racial harassment were not reported to senior management. Staff felt that they were expected to ignore harassment by patients in particular, because it was considered 'unprofessional' to be upset by racist comments. They also reported that they had little confidence in the benefits of reporting incidents to managers. On the few occasions when management were reported as having tried to tackle the problem, the response was regarded as inadequate. Several minority ethnic nurses reported actually being replaced by white nurses when racist patients had refused to be cared for by them. This has the effect of 'rewarding' the discriminatory behaviour of patients and undermining the minority ethnic nurse. Other writers have suggested that ethnic minority nurses are reluctant to complain because they do not feel that they will be listened to or supported by their managers and that indeed, they are fearful of losing their jobs (Healy 1996).

As Beishon *et al.* (1995: 134) have argued, 'Racial harassment in the workplace affects the performance of an organisation by creating a climate of isolation and hostility, and this can ultimately detract from the development of an effective and efficient health service'. Despite this, however, policies to address the problem of racial harassment and victimisation only covered harassment involving colleagues and not patients, although the latter was by far the bigger problem.

Equal opportunities policies

Formal equal opportunities (EO) policies are almost universal in NHS trusts, yet the evidence shows that while there have been

some excellent initiatives in a small number of NHS organizations, many trusts are failing to carry out even the basic ethnic
monitoring functions required by the NHS Executive (MSF
1997). Progress in formulating and especially in implementing
and evaluating equal opportunitiy policies has been slow and
patchy (Law 1996). A minority of authorities and trusts have
made some significant efforts, but many have failed to put
formal policies into practice.

In October 1997 the NHS Equal Opportunities Unit commissioned a survey of EO policies, practices and monitoring in
the NHS throughout England. This shows that while most
trusts have a general policy statement which covers equal
opportunities in employment, only 59 per cent have policies on
harassment by patients (Hurstfield 1998). The overall survey
and case studies in this research show a continuing gap between
formal policies and their effective implementation, as well as
highlighting poor communication of policies to staff. Policies
were poorly disseminated and inconsistently implemented. Consistent weaknesses in the collection of ethnic monitoring data
were reported in many trusts, while complete data on recruitment, promotions, redundancies, dismissals and training was
available for only a minority. Good practice in a small minority
of trusts is evident, alongside the widespread failure of many to
develop and evaluate equal opportunities policies. Many trusts
seem to have gone little further than the collection of ethnic
monitoring data, and some, as the MSF research shows, have
not even achieved this.

The examination of equal opportunities policies and practice
in the PSI study of nursing found very significant gaps between
written policies identified by senior and general managers and
the actual practices undertaken in the workplace. Senior management expressed a firm commitment to equal opportunities
but had either failed to follow through formal policies into
specific objectives such as implementing appraisal schemes or
examining the allocation of training opportunities. Middle and
line managers (such as ward sisters) were often unclear about
what the equal opportunities policy was and how they were supposed to undertake their responsibilities within it.

The research found

little evidence if any that those responsible for formulating a policy were analysing the outcomes in ways which would help them decide whether it was being carried out, or whether it was having the desired effect. Quite a lot of monitoring information was *collected* (information was recorded on forms and sent to the personnel department); only some of it was ever *processed* (in the sense that tables were produced); hardly any of it was *analysed* and *assessed* (in the sense of helping to take decisions about future action). (Beishon *et al.* 1995: 228, emphasis in original)

Minority ethnic nurses in leadership roles

Despite considerable barriers, there are many minority ethnic nurses who have negotiated the obstacles in their nursing careers and achieved leadership positions. Research carried out by Mayor (1996) has investigated the career experiences of leading minority ethnic nurses using oral 'topical career' histories/ biography and supplementary questionnaire. In-depth interviews were conducted with 88 informants (28 males and 60 females). Seventeen categorized themselves as Black African, 37 as African-Caribbean and 34 as Asian. Of these, four were British born. The participants were employed at clinical grade H or above or at equivalent levels in related employment sectors such as nursing education, research or policy development. The research provides rich insights into the processes of 'becoming careerists'; the factors which support career mobility; the development of support networks and the staying power of these leading minority nurses.

The interviews revealed a range of ways in which the respondents critically analysed the career choices open to them as they entered the labour market. Influences of ethnicity, gender and social class (Sokoloff 1992; Mirza 1992), access to education and cultural capital (Bourdieu 1993) on the individuals choice of career, their perceived position in the labour market and subsequent opportunities for career mobility indicate the complexities negotiated at a personal level.

The research confirms many of the difficulties experienced by the 'overseas' recruits discussed earlier in the chapter. For example, despite having appropriate entry qualifications, 33 of the informants were require to take the GNC test on arrival in the UK. One informant was subjected to a heavy inquisition about her knowledge of the test procedure and asked to re-sit it because she achieved a 100 per cent pass. Eighteen informants began their nursing careers in the enrolled nurse stream even though 13 of these met the criteria for the registered stream pre and post the GNC test. Transfer from enrolled to registered stream during training was successful for three informants. All three had used similar strategies as levers to negotiate transfer, that is, each had either informed or threatened to inform their sponsors (in their home countries) and made sure that officers in the relevant UK based embassy/high commission knew of their disadvantage.

Many informants referred to negative experiences in their early career as a spur, with the 'I'll show them' syndrome coming into play. Unlike other research, these informants are not clustered in Cinderella services such as mental health or elderly care or delivery of services targeted at minority clients. Several informants cited examples of the way in which their language skills were widely used or essential in their job, for example in health visiting or midwifery care, but regrettably these skills were not usually recognized in their job specification and grading for the post. The inadequate provision of interpreters in the NHS means that staff are often called upon to act as *ad hoc* interpreters. While many staff are willing to do this, it does mean that often they are taken away from their own duties. All informants recognized the interplay of ethnic identity, gender, social class and organizational structures as affecting their career development.

Research literature emphasizes the role of mentoring and networks in career development (Davidson 1997; Wedderburn Tate 1998). In this study, mentoring was infrequent and brief and almost always carried out by white men or women. With hind sight, virtually all informants were able to recognize 'mentoring like inputs' from line managers, peers, nurse tutors or people in other professions but the stark reality of transient, brief episodes, often unfocused or unrelated to the broader context suggests that these individuals succeeded without having had recourse to what is considered as a vital component of career development. Many of the participants mentioned the support from partners, families, friends, church seniors, former school teachers as well as informal peer support networks which operated outside the work place. Their conclusion was that this support was vital to them for assessing their progress, testing out aspirations and ideas and as a safety net when things went awry. Though membership of special interest groups at national or local level was instrumental in reducing professional isolation and promoting the opportunity for contact and sharing, these are viewed as an 'add on' to the support received from family and friends. A study of minority ethnic managers in local government also suggested that these individuals benefited from mentoring, shadowing and networking and suggested setting targets for achieving greater numbers from minority ethnic groups in local government and the NHS (Wedderburn Tate 1998).

The future for equal opportunities in nursing

What is required to take forward the equal opportunities agenda in the NHS? Several research reports in the past ten or more years have produced comprehensive proposals and recommendations. The PSI report (Beishon *et al.* 1995) contains a list of recommendations to make the NHS a more friendly environment for minority ethnic staff. Trusts, it is argued, need to

- effectively communicate equal opportunities policies to everyone in the organization concerned;
- provide appropriate training for staff responsible for the implementation of policy;
- devise a process of enforcement of policy;
- make everyone in the organization responsible for dealing with racial harassment by means of a carefully thought out campaign to convince staff that racial harassment is an unacceptable feature of NHS life.

It could be argued that what is missing is the political determination to enforce existing policies. The Labour Government elected in 1997 has, like its predecessor, expressed a commitment to improving the position of ethnic minorities in the NHS. The NHS has signed up to the Leadership Challenge, launched by the Commission for Racial Equality in 1997, which aims to ensure that companies throughout Britain see racial equality as a key component of their business. This is very much in line with the 'business case' for equal opportunities which is the approach taken by both Conservative and Labour governments in recent years.

Social justice arguments for equal opportunities policies are important for the NHS as a major public sector employer. However, appeals to fairness and equity do not appear to have taken policies very far in many cases. The 'business case' for equal opportunities refers to arguments relating to organizational self-interest. Organizational self-interest might be served in several ways by the proper implementation of EO initiatives. For example, it could be argued that EO policies might help to recruit and retain ethnic minority nurses which would help to address current labour shortages. There is a recruitment and retention crisis in the NHS amongst nurses in particular and the potential pool of recruits among minority ethnic groups in the UK is seen by some as one part of the solution to this (Buchan 1998). Since nursing remains a relatively low paid profession there are clear dangers in seeing this as a slot to be filled by ethnic minorities, leading to further marginalization.

Equal opportunities policies are significant therefore, since, it could be argued, minority groups must see progress on reducing racial inequality if they are to be attracted to nursing as a career. However, before minority ethnic nurses can be employed they must be recruited to *training*. As we have seen, there is little evidence that educational institutions are adequately addressing this issue, with relatively few colleges either taking special measures to attract ethnic minority recruits or to adequately support them once recruited (Gerrish *et al.* 1996). The authors of the ENB-commissioned research project on recruitment and selection of minority ethnic groups into nurse education have recommended that the ENB (or its successor) encourage educational institutions to adopt and implement policies which commit them to diversity in the student population and the equitable treatment of applicants in their selection processes. The importance of establishing links with minority ethnic community organizations is also stressed (Iganski *et al.* 1998).

An additional reason frequently advanced as part of the 'business case' for equal opportunities is that the employment of larger numbers of workers from minority ethnic backgrounds would have considerable benefits for the effective delivery of health care to minority ethnic communities. However, there are certain questionable assumptions built into this argument. The NHS is already the largest employer of ethnic minorities in Britain. Ward (1993) has argued that the NHS provides the strongest case to refute the argument that opening up an organization to 'black and ethnic minority' staff *inevitably* leads to change in favour of ethnic minority users. It is, he argues, precisely in those areas where black professionals are concentrated (psychiatry, geriatrics) that the system is regarded as perhaps the least appropriate for minority ethnic users. The employment of ethnic minority workers is desirable for many reasons, but it is not in itself a guarantee of improved service delivery (Culley 1997). It cannot be assumed that minority ethnic health professionals who have undergone traditional training will have the necessary skills to work in a culturally competent way with all minority groups (Gerrish *et al.* 1996). The additional skills which some members of the minority ethnic workforce bring to their jobs (such as languages additional to English) are often taken for granted and unrewarded by employers (Beishon *et al.* 1995).

There are, however, two major disincentives to the effective implementation of EO policies in the NHS. The first concerns financial costs. The 'good business sense' argument may well be problematic for the NHS, at a time when resources are tight. Many NHS trusts are in severe financial difficulties and have many other pressures on expenditure. Against this however, it could be argued that the potential costs of not taking issues such as racial harassment seriously could be significant since legal cases brought against employers who fail to act to prevent this could result in substantial awards to staff. Employers are potentially liable for any act of harassment committed by employees in the course of their employment and recent cases suggest that employers are also under a duty to protect their employees from harassment by clients while doing their job. The second issue concerns the relative weight which is likely to be given to the equal opportunities agenda in the context of other major changes in NHS structures and operations such as the development of primary care groups and trusts, trust mergers, and the new quality agenda. It is quite possible that under the pressure of such major changes equal opportunities issues will receive less attention, unless managers ensure that an equality perspective is an integral part of these developments.

In addition to possible pragmatic reasons for the lack of consistent progress in the NHS, several writers have questioned equal opportunities policies in a more fundamental way, although it is not possible to review the arguments in any detail here (Jewson and Mason 1986; Jenkins and Solomos 1989; Rattansi 1992; Law 1996). It is possible to argue that equal opportunities policies are fundamentally flawed in the way they construct the problem of racial equality and therefore, even if fully implemented would not necessarily produce 'equity' in terms of outcomes.

> The current focus is on helping ethnic minorities, the disabled and women compete 'on equal terms' with white non-disabled men for jobs which have been shaped around the typical circumstances of white, able bodied men, within organisations where the culture, norms, values, notions of merit, formal and informal structures all reflect the attributes, needs, work and life patterns of the typical white non-disabled male. (Dickens 1994: 287–8)

A major criticism of EO policies, then, is the fact that they are not designed to challenge the definitions of normality or acceptability which are used as the basis for racist exclusion. They may allow gains or achievements for some individuals – and they may allow these gains to be consolidated, but the basic template remains the same.

Conclusion

This chapter has examined the historical background to the contribution of minority ethnic nurses to the NHS, arguing that there has been evidence of disadvantage and discrimination since the beginnings of the service. It has examined the research evidence which shows the difficulties which many minority ethnic nurses still face in applying for nurse training and in the course of their studies. It has examined equal opportunities policies and argued that although there is a long history of efforts to combat racial discrimination in the NHS, policies and initiatives have been piecemeal and fragmented, with very little monitoring of targets and few penalties for non-compliance.

In 1998, the Labour Secretary of State for Health outlined a strategy for the NHS which includes

● efforts to increase the representation of ethnic minorities on trust boards
● improvements in the level of ethnic monitoring
● funding a range of 'positive action' projects
● the launch of an NHS Equality Awards scheme.

The government has funded, by way of the Equal Opportunities Unit, a national programme called Positively Diverse to assist health and social care organizations to recruit, retain and develop a workforce representative of a multicultural society. This is set within the context of the new human resource strategy set out in the document *Working Together: Securing a quality workforce for the NHS* (Department of Health 1998a). The quality of the human resource function is often a major barrier to effective implementation of equal opportunities strategies and the human resource function in many NHS trusts is often weak, particularly in relation to the power exercised by professional groups generally and the medical profession in particular (Salter 1998).

In late 1998 the government also announced a plan to tackle racial harassment in the NHS, whereby all employers are to be set targets to reduce incidents of racial harassment (Department of Health 1998b). This has been built upon in a document produced as part of the 'modernization' agenda introduced in 2000. *The Vital Connection* (Department of Health 2000), sets out a strategic framework for action during 2000–04 to improve recruitment from under-represented groups, to ensure that the NHS is a fair employer and to ensure that the NHS uses its resources to make a difference to disadvantaged sections of local communities. Each NHS organization will be required to publish an 'equality statement' as part of its annual report, setting out how they are taking forward a commitment to equality. The government plan to establish a core set of equality indicators and national standards covering issues of ethnicity, gender, disability and age. Objectives are to be taken forward within the performance management framework of *Working Together*.

There are then, some hopeful signs of progress, but it is clear that there is still a long way to go before racial harassment and discrimination are a thing of the past for Britain's minority ethnic nurses.

11 Caribbean nurses and racism in the National Health Service

Lorraine Culley, Simon Dyson, Silvia Ham-Ying and Wendy Young

Introduction

In this chapter we briefly review some of the major contributions to sociological analyses of the professions, and the critique of professionalism as a positive project for the development of nursing. The chapter then recounts the recent postwar history of Caribbean-born nurses in the National Health Service (NHS), charting the labour shortages which helped to stimulate their arrival; their relative invisibility in terms of documentation of numbers, experiences and career progress; and the challenges which they faced. This is followed by a discussion of some of the findings from interviews carried out by the authors with fourteen first level nurses and midwives who were part of the postwar migration to Britain from the Caribbean and who have each contributed the majority of their working lives to the NHS.

Sociology and the professions

There has been a considerable debate regarding the nature of professionalism and its relevance to nursing (Porter 1998; Wilkinson and Miers 1999), though issues of 'race' or ethnicity rarely feature in sociological debates on professionalism. Early sociological work on the professions was dominated by an approach which took the form of a listing of traits which were said to characterize professions such as a long period of training, self-regulation, autonomy and altruism (putting the needs of clients before the needs of professionals themselves). Medicine is usually regarded as the archetypal profession according to this perspective. Functionalist theorists identified professions such as medicine and law as being highly rewarded by virtue of the possession of scarce skills that were needed for society as a whole to function smoothly (Goode 1960).

These naïve early accounts have been challenged in a number of ways. They are regarded as accepting professionals' own idealized account of their activities at face value and as failing to see the negative impact which professionalism might have on clients and on other occupational groups. *Interactionist* sociologists such as Becker *et al.* (1961) began, through close observational studies, to examine the behaviour of professionals (especially doctors). Contrary to trait theorists they found unexpectedly low standards of moral behaviour and evidence of disdain for clients. Freidson (1970) and Parkin (1979) saw professions as occupations who have successfully used a strategy of professionalization to their own advantage (see Porter 1998). It is argued, for example, that in controlling access to medical training doctors are able to create themselves as a scarce resource, reap the benefits of large financial rewards and maintain control over the terms and conditions under which they work. Moreover, since doctors themselves also largely control the regulation of the medical profession, they are judge and jury on their own behaviour, and so lack public accountability. In this view acting professionally may involve manoeuvring to gain status, financial reward and other privileges. At the same time the professions are able to manipulate an altruistic image of themselves through the maintenance of a professional ideology of public service (Johnson 1972).

Where does nursing stand in these analyses? The over-reliance on medicine as a model led commentators such as Etzioni (1969) to talk of nursing as a 'semi-profession', relatively lacking in control over working conditions, control of access to the occupation's training and relatively lacking in a distinctive body of disciplinary knowledge. Interestingly the spirit, if not the derogatory term, of this type of analysis appears to have been taken up by nurses themselves (Porter 1992). Hence Witz (1992) notes the increased emphasis on credentialism (getting paper qualifications) as part of the process which nursing has apparently adopted in an attempt to be recognized as a full profession. In this respect, some Caribbean migrants were ahead of their time in that they had credentials at least comparable to those of whites, having experienced a traditional British curriculum through the colonial education system. The increased emphasis on a research base for nursing, the proliferation of nursing models, the implementation of the nursing process and the migration into higher education can be seen as part of the striving for professional status and the expectation of financial rewards (Porter 1992; Miers 1999). However, as Porter (1998) has argued, this strategy fails to take into account nursing's relationship with other occupational groups, especially medicine. This issue is examined in some detail in the work of Davies (1995) where the significance of gender is highlighted. Davies (1995) argues that nursing is not a profession but the *means* by which medicine becomes and maintains its position as a profession. The professional autonomy of doctors is only possible through ignoring the work of other, predominantly female, occupational groups.

More recent debate has then, challenged the essentially benign view of professions and professionalization and challenged the appropriateness of occupations such as nursing striving for professional status (Salvage 1985). The power of professionals has also been subjected to concerted challenge from politicians and consumer groups (Gabe *et al.* 1994; Wilkinson and Miers 1999). At the same time, although writers have considered the gendered nature of professionalism (Davies 1995) and the significance of an analysis of gender relations to professionalising strategies in nursing, there has been no corresponding effort to locate the significance of ethnicity in such strategies. There is research evidence concerning the existence of 'racial' discrimination within medicine and nursing (Beishon *et al.* 1995; Esmail *et al.* 1995, 1998), but this has not been extensively discussed in the context of professionalisation.

One consequence of taking the rhetoric of professionalism at face value is that it undermines the possibility of an adequate assessment of racism and nursing. Racial stereotyping of clients and staff from minority ethnic groups by some nurses and midwives remains a problem (Bowler 1993a, b; Porter 1993; Bowes and Domokos 1996). The traditional view of professionalism includes the assumption that professionals have a universalistic orientation (Parsons 1951) in which, for example, nurses achieve ideal standards of care by virtue of 'treating everyone the same'. However, this ignores the different social, economic and cultural location of patients and clients. In addition, professional ideology portrays professionals as people of whom a high standard of moral behaviour is expected. Racist behaviour by professionals is so contrary to the ideals of behaviour enshrined in codes of conduct that it is more difficult to accept that racism may nevertheless inform professional practices (Porter 1993). An analysis of racisms, and an analysis of professionalism, will both be limited if conceived of only in terms of individual behaviour rather than as part of wider social relations.

It is because of the importance of considering these wider circumstances that before considering the experiences of Caribbean-born nurses and midwives in the health service and their responses to racism, we need to describe the processes of migration that brought them to Britain in the first instance and the social profile of the respondents to our interviews.

Caribbean migration and nursing in the NHS

The period of postwar immigration between the 1948 British Nationality Act and the Commonwealth Immigrants Act 1962 expanded rather than created the presence of black people in the UK (Fryer 1984; Ramdin 1987; Small 1994). During the Second World War, Britain actively recruited labour from the Caribbean to help with the war effort in the factories (Fryer 1984) and the armed services (Gilroy 1987; Harris 1993).

The British Nationality Act 1948 gave Commonwealth citizens special immigration status, with the right to freely enter, work and settle with their families. However, this migration peaked in the early 1960s and was effectively over by 1973, by which time the Caribbean-born population of Britain was about 550,000 (Peach 1986). The Commonwealth Immigrants Act 1962 established legal controls of the entry of Commonwealth citizens for the first time and this restriction on primary immigration was extended by both Labour and Conservative governments in 1968 and 1971 respectively. The Immigration Act 1971 effectively ended all new primary immigration from the so-called 'New Commonwealth' (Mason 1995).

Labour shortages existed in the newly formed National Health Service, with an estimated shortfall of 54,000 nurses in 1949 (Harris 1993). Previously hospitals had relied on Irish workers to make up shortfalls in staffing levels as white British workers were, on the whole, reluctant to work the long hours and shifts for low pay. However, postwar there was a noticeable reduction of Irish immigration. Overseas nurses played a significant role in filling the gaps in the delivery of the service. Substantial numbers of Caribbean-born men and women entered the NHS from the early 1950s (Doyal et al. 1980).

Recruitment campaigns were carried out throughout the Commonwealth, with senior British nurses visiting the countries in pursuit of labour (Baxter 1988). However, direct recruitment mainly affected Barbados, where just under a quarter of the emigrants in 1960 left on sponsorship schemes.

The absence of comprehensive ethnic monitoring makes any estimate of the extent of the contribution of Caribbean-born workers difficult, but available evidence suggests a substantial concentration of black migrants in ancillary work such as domestic, catering, cleaning and maintenance jobs. Nevertheless, many Caribbean migrants also entered nursing. By 1971, it was estimated that there were over 15,000 'overseas nurses' in the NHS. Thomas and Morton-Williams (1972) found that 9 per cent of hospital nurses were born overseas (of these half were from the West Indies, and a quarter each from Africa and Asia) and that 'immigrants' were 20 per cent of pupil nurses, 15 per cent of midwives and 14 per cent of student nurses. This study identified an under-representation of overseas nurses in senior grades and found that overseas nurses were more likely to be found in the less popular and less prestigious specialities such as geriatric and mental health nursing. The number of Caribbean-born recruits declined from 1970 and by the mid-1980s had virtually ceased.

Despite the presence of a large proportion of ethnic minority nurses, there was little research or data on how they had fared in the NHS (Akinsanya 1988). It was not until after the enactment of the Race Relations Act 1976 that the issue of possible racial discrimination in the service could be legally addressed. Moreover, it was not until 1992 that a large-scale national study of the careers of ethnic minority nurses was carried out (Beishon *et al.* 1995). Evidence from the early years is fragmentary, yet suggests that many nurses suffered racial discrimination (Thomas and Morton-Williams 1972; Hicks 1982; Baxter 1988; Ward 1993). Indeed, small-scale qualitative studies paint a very bleak picture, highlighting difficulties that these nurses face at all stages of their careers (Baxter 1988; Lee-Cunin 1989).

In a period of increased difficulty in recruitment to the health services (George 1994) people of Caribbean descent have been less likely to enter nursing. While there are calls for racism to be challenged in recruitment to the health service (King's Fund 1990), and in the working environment of nurses (Beishon *et al.* 1995) we know little about the experiences of Caribbean-born nurses and midwives some of whom have contributed their entire working lives to the NHS.

The respondents

This chapter draws on interviews with eight female and six male respondents all of whom were first level nurses or midwives. The first/second level distinction is no longer embedded in nurse education, but until the 1980s, first level nurses had a longer period of training and undertook a wider range of responsibilities than second level nurses who worked under their guidance (Nurses, Midwives and Health Visitors Rules 1983). Many Caribbean-born nurses were channelled into the second level, state enrolled nursing. They were also heavily over-represented in the less prestigious specialities of psychiatric and 'mental handicap' nursing. All six of the men and three of the women are qualified and have worked as mental health nurses. (Of these, four of the men and one of the women were also dual qualified in general nursing.) The remaining five female respondents trained as general nurses and subsequently three specialized in midwifery and had registered midwife qualifications. Six of the fourteen (four men and two women) had achieved fairly high level positions within nursing, as nursing officer, nurse manager or senior clinical nurse, before retirement. This level of occupational achievement marks our interviewees out as different from the respondents in Fenton (1988) and Lee-Cunin (1989) and may explain why their reported experiences are mixed rather than overwhelmingly negative.

Few early Caribbean migrants had intentions to settle permanently in Britain (Glass 1960; Patterson 1965; Daniel 1968; Lawrence 1974) and this was the case with the majority of our respondents (see Table 11.1). The fact that their original intentions had not been carried through seemed to be viewed with a certain amount of resignation and of humour rather than regret. The prospect of better opportunities coupled with a lack of good employment prospects at home had been a major impetus for migration and entry to nurse training was relatively easy at a time of labour shortage. Several were taken on almost immediately upon arrival in Britain and worked on the wards until they were able to join a cohort of entrants to begin formal training.

Return migration to the Caribbean has always been significant (Peach 1991). However, at the end of their working lives the majority of our respondents see no real permanent place for themselves in their islands of origin and/or feel tied by strong relationships with family (especially children) and friends. Most have been fortunate in being able to return to visit the Caribbean on a very regular basis over the years and this contact is valued.

Negative experiences, professionalism and racism

Our interviews with the Caribbean nurses suggest that a naïve understanding of professionalism as a set of positive traits is inadequate in at least five ways.

(1) It ignores the relationship of nursing to other occupational groups, most obviously to the profession of medicine.

[. . .] it didn't occur to me to think in terms of being a doctor. Because in those days you just thought of doctors being male, and in our

Table 11.1 Profile of the respondents.

Respondent	Position	Age at interview	Arrival in UK	NHS service (years)	Total service (years)
A	Home manager	72	1957	18	34
B	Nurse manager	64	1955	34	34
C	Midwife	70	1958	31	31
D	Nurse manager	52	1962	31	31
E	Midwife	61	1959	35	35
F	Nursing officer	64	1954	39	39
G	Manager	60	1957	35	40
H	Senior nurse	56	1960	34	37
I	Nursing officer	59	1959	34	34
J	Senior sister	59	1956	39	39
K	Senior nurse	51	1966	27	32
L	Home manager	52	1966	20	32
M	Staff nurse	62	1960	25	30
N	Nursing sister	54	1963	12	28
		Mean = 59.7		Mean = 29.6	Mean = 34.0

country anyway they were all sort of white males anyway. (Respondent H)

The successful occupational closure of the medical profession is based on the ascribed characteristics of the competitors to doctors. Thus both in gender terms and in terms of ethnicity our respondent had developed a mindset in which she excludes herself from a medical career on the basis that she is Caribbean and female and that doctors are white and male.

(2) Analyzing professionalism as a set of traits also ignores the wider societal contexts of power. Employment in the health service involves contradictions for our interviewees. On the one hand it is, as we shall see, the source of racisms of white staff and white patients. On the other hand the institutional setting provides a refuge from certain wider societal racisms.

> The other thing that cushioned people like me who came to work in the hospital service . . . there were such things as nursing homes . . . so we didn't have the trauma of having to look for accommodation and being rebuked and rebuffed and discarded. (Respondent G)

(3) The trait approach also assumes that professional status is a state of being and not an ongoing process. But professionalized occupations often have a long process of qualifying stages involving various processes of socialization, in the case of nursing from student nurse to qualified nurse for example.

> Do you know the charge nurses . . . they all sat . . . over there. They never said a word to you and this would go on for six weeks. All new students were ignored by charge nurses for six weeks . . . We had a very small charge nurse who would tell us almost everything and said, 'How you getting on the ward?' and we said, 'Fine', and he said, 'Such and such your charge nurse, is he talking to you now?'. And I said, 'Yes, what do you mean?' and he said, 'Six weeks pass. Charge nurses don't talk to students under six weeks'. In truth, and that was true, six weeks to the day that we were patted on the shoulder and offered cigarettes and things like that. And before that nothing. Funny world we live in. Very strange, very strange. (Respondent A)

The uneasiness which Respondent A experiences could have been attributed by him to racist attitudes. Instead the incident has been interpreted as a consequence of the occupational hierarchy which applied irrespective of ethnic status. It is seen as being part of the occupational socialization of nurses in which as student nurses they are fair game to be treated badly and ignored and in which acceptance comes only when the transition from new student to established student status has been made.

(4) To think of professionals as naturally having certain characteristics also ignores the existence of continuing formal hierarchies within occupations which describe themselves as professions. In the case of nursing, staff nurses, charge nurses, ward sisters and matrons are (or were for the period of time we are describing) each located within a strict hierarchy of power and status. Even after qualification the rigid hierarchy within nursing continued. Once again, the feeling of being oppressed through power relationships could have been experienced by the Caribbean-born nurses simply as racism, but was in fact seen more as a product of an extremely hierarchical division of labour.

> . . . I'm looking back now and trying to find a kindly sister and I don't think I can find one. I think they're all fairly sort of . . . brutal really and very hierarchical and do-as-you're-told and so on. So I think if there is racism being sort of dished out to me then it was all part and parcel of a very, a fairly harsh regime really. (Respondent H)

In this account by Respondent H racism is allowed to remain as a possible explanation. It is not clear if the weight of oppression was such that from the point of view of the respondent it hardly mattered whether or not it had a racial dimension.

(5) There are many other informal relations of power which cross-cut these internal divisions within professions. These include different relations between staff and colleagues and between staff and patients. These also include relations of age, and of gender.

For example, the experience of being ascribed a lowly status in an occupational hierarchy in common with others (in other words the very opposite of professionalism as an ideology, but very much how professional occupations actually work) is found to partially protect against the effects of racist clients.

> The funny thing about living in nursing homes in those days is that you actually develop something like on board ship, camaraderie,

you're all in it together. We were all low paid, we all had to do the same mucky old jobs and so, I mean people, we weren't singled out for those . . . if you did the worst job it was according to how junior you were as opposed to where you came from. So I have to say I didn't meet much neg/ There was the odd negative . . . my first interaction with patients there were the odd negative situations. But I think really, as you mature, or are maturing, I think you learn to, not so much ignore that, but cope with it and don't see it as a threat. (Respondent G)

The negative experiences of racism are acknowledged in this extract but downplayed because (i) there was a camaraderie (presumably including white colleagues) to working together in adversity; (ii) negative experiences in this instance were from patients not colleagues; and (iii) the respondent himself adopts a naïve concept of professionalism in that coping with racism is thought of by the respondent as a matter of personal growth.

So far we have looked at how hierarchies and ascribed status relations disorganize experiences of racisms. But negative experiences may be associated with gender relationships as well as ethnic relations.

Yes, she was a white girl that got the Sister's post. And I learned after this, because of the interrelationship with one of the senior managers, the usual thing (laughs). I did not know this at the time (laughing). (Respondent D)

Here, Respondent D attributes thwarted prospects for promotion to sexual relations between a white manager and a white nurse, and although this is acknowledged as corrupt and as an example of generalized gender power relations ('the usual thing'), it is presented as a individualized piece of bad luck and timing. Therefore her initial suspicions of racism are implied to have been mistaken in retrospect. It was immoral and unfair, but it was sexism at work rather than racism.

In other instances negative encounters are also ascribed to relations based on age, either the age of the patient, or the age of the staff. In the following excerpt, it is unclear whether the patient does not want to be lifted by the male Caribbean nurse because of his ethnicity, because he is male or for some other reason. It is suggested however, that this attitude on behalf of the patient might be something to do with her generation, and that a refusal to be helped because of perceived blackness or maleness would be relatively less likely to come from a younger patient.

> Some of them (patients) still, especially the older type and they still say 'Oh, I don't want you to lift me up; you know and like everything' ... I said, OK, I'll get somebody else to lift them if they ask me to do it. But again that was over a period of time they sort of came round, they see your face and recognize that I was a nurse. I think this is something that people don't always realize that older peoples always recognize a young lady or a woman as a nurse, they never recognize a guy um even now even in this day and age. (Respondent F)

And so the nature of the discrimination is felt by the speaker to be one of a generation gap in understanding that a man could be a nurse. However, one could argue that racism is at work because the patient does not appear to recognize that a Caribbean person could be qualified (because if they were not a nurse, then in the eyes of the older patient they presumably could only be an unqualified auxiliary, assuming they would not have objected to a doctor lifting them).

Another element of age-related discrimination concerns the age of and processes of compulsory redundancies dressed up as early retirements.

> It wasn't the going that bothers me, it was the manner in which I was forced to go, out. I did get a letter ... thanking me for my loyalty, but that's not the point. I don't want to do anything in fact I'm happy that I don't have to go to work. I'm just peeved about the way that I was expected to end it. .... But I can't say this happened to me because I'm black, because it happened to others as well that weren't black. I mean maybe I could say it happened to me because of my age (Respondent I)

Here, Respondent I reflects somewhat bitterly on early retirement. There is a clear recognition that this is happening to white colleagues of the same age as part of the multiple NHS reorganizations, and is cause enough for legitimate bitterness at the belittlement of their occupational contribution. Whether there was racial discrimination at work is felt to be impossible to judge from an individual perspective, and the implication is that one would have to examine the patterns to make such a case. The poor quality of ethnic monitoring in the NHS suggests these patterns may remain hidden. The resignation in the account of the respondent may mean they themselves are resigned to such patterns never being discovered.

In summary, the experiences of Caribbean-born nurses are understandable neither in terms of naïve accounts of professionalism, nor in terms of simply describing negative incidents in terms of racisms. Their reported experiences are also marked by relations of student and occupational status, by gender relations and by relations of age and generation as well as racism. It is important to remember as well that as first level nurses and midwives their working lives may have been differently experienced compared to the extreme adversities reported by nurses in Baxter (1988) or Lee-Cunin (1989), or by Caribbean migrants from a range of occupations interviewed by Fenton (1988).

'Backstage racisms'

Porter (1993) introduces the notion of racisms occurring 'backstage' when the mask of professional relations is let slip, when nurses are on breaks or in other informal circumstances. The important point about this for our purposes here is that it means that racisms must be considered as structuring experiences of the Caribbean nurses *even when those racisms are not observable in any immediate interactions* (see Porter 1998). Early research undertaken by Lawrence (1974: 52) confirms this view since he found that discrimination in employment was relatively covert compared to the open hostility faced by Caribbean migrants in other areas of public life. It is important to remember, though, that the Caribbean nurses do not themselves necessarily have access to these 'backstage racisms'. Thus they may be faced with situations where they are conscious of racism as actually or potentially informing encounters, but where they are unsure of its precise role in a given situation.

> Because when I qualified, when I got my general, I recall going to see the chief male nurse. I told him, I want to discuss the future, what my situation would be like if I stayed on, and he said, 'You come to ask me for advice, I will say to you get out', he said, 'there's nothing here for you'. Well I didn't run off and say his views are racist. I just took his advice and I decided, well, I'm going and try elsewhere. (Respondent B)

It is not clear whether the experience evidences racism in promotion (there's nothing for you here because I, the chief nurse, am a racist) or whether the advice is a realistic appraisal of a racist society (there's nothing for you here because other people here are racist). It could also be the case that the apparently realistic appraisal of a racist society by the chief nurse is actually a more sophisticated and self-protecting racism in operation (I'm using other people's racism as an excuse to encourage you to leave but really I want you to leave as well).

Furthermore, the nurses may consciously or unconsciously structure their own experiences to take account of previous or anticipated racisms.

> I worked in highly intensive areas [smiles] because the patients don't argue with you. They're too ill to argue with you [laughing]. So maybe I don't get the full brunt of what patients on big wards, or any wards for that matter, who are not so well . . . to, to, to, erm criticise you too much. The majority of my senior time has been in specialised care. And probably that's why I think, they are more or less, the relatives are so appreciative, of what you can, of what you do to them, that I don't get time, I don't have the experience of *pettiness* [pettiness said with contempt] you know. . . . I don't know if you understand what I'm saying. (Respondent J)

The implication is that the racism of both the patients and relatives is moderated in an intensive care situation – patients because they are too ill and dependent and relatives because racism is temporarily suspended in extreme situations where their relative may die. This is presented by Respondent J as an experience which is unlike the more overt racism she felt she had endured elsewhere and indeed a motivating factor for her to enter and remain within that speciality.

In summary, Caribbean nurses had to deal not only with overt racism where the negative experience was very clear but they were also faced by many ambiguous situations in which it is not clear whether the hostility they faced was attributable to racism. Experiences of racism may also have affected the types of work they felt secure in undertaking.

Moral resistance to racisms

However, the respondents also recounted episodes where they themselves clearly felt racisms overtly directed at them. But this does not mean that these instances were ignored. Unwelcome statuses ascribed on the basis of racism are not passively accepted, but may be challenged, modified, or otherwise used in more positive ways in the creation of identities (Modood *et al.* 1994).

We can identify three dimensions to the responses of the Caribbean nurses to racisms. First, there is the recognition that it *is* racism (rather than other relations of power) that they are experiencing. Second, there is the contrast to the cultured image of white people the respondents had carried with them from the Caribbean. And third, emerging from this contrast, there is the construction of a sense of their own moral worth.

The confrontation with undesirable qualities in others is shown in the negative experiences specifically attributed wholly or partly to racisms. Here are some examples of what the Caribbean nurses were subjected to:

Physical violence: One of our respondents was, in the 1950s, called across the road from the hospital and punched violently in the face – what we would now clearly call a racist attack.

Racialism: Name-calling (monkey noises in outpatients; references to recent emergence from the jungle; enquiries about living in mud huts).

Direct racial discrimination: Patients refusing their attempts to care for them, colleagues refusing to sit next to black staff or to work under black staff; white colleagues refusing to return everyday pleasantries.

Indirect racial discrimination: For example, having to take additional entrance tests, disproportionately not receiving official rewards or being refused choices in work patterns afforded to others.

Racial stereotyping: Staff and patients stereotyping Caribbean people as always happy-go-lucky; having magical powers of healing; or being knowledgeable about tropical diseases.

Unlike the discriminators, the Caribbean nurses often specifically referred to 'keeping an open mind', not pre-judging others, not judging a whole group on the basis of the behaviour of a minority and so on.

The second dimension in the response to racism can be seen in the contrast between colonial images of white people and the realities of some white behaviours and cultures.

> . . . you know when you see an English person in the West Indies with bright coloured clothing looking clean and erm, well-shaved and rather arrogant and full of themselves, and you almost begin to believe that they're better than yourself. Well when I arrive(d) at Southampton myself I saw rather drab looking men in long gabardine coats, um, smoking woodbines and looking er, half starved almost, you know. . . . I met some chappies from very good backgrounds in Barbados, walking the streets of Birmingham in tears 'cos they were being, 'cos they were seeing you know, accommodation advertised and then they would go along and the minute they saw they were black they would say, oh sorry its gone . . . we really believe(d) that thing about, you know, fairness in Britain and erm, and that we were really part of this thing called the Empire and the Commonwealth and that, and that we would be welcome. Because we thought, why would people come and invite you to come to their place, if they didn't want to treat you well. (Respondent G)

Our respondents recounted occasions where they felt *some* white people they met had behaved in ways they considered to be aggressive, unfriendly and discriminatory. Sometimes this was also how the Caribbean nurses felt that white 'friends' they had come to trust were also behaving. Against this backdrop, it is easier to see the emergence of a third dimension in responding to racism. This takes the form of resisting racism through strong moral frameworks, for example, self-consciously behaving well in the face of others behaving badly. Two illustrations of this are provided here. In the first example, the tolerance shown others is conceived as maturity, with the black person as responsible adult and the white person as immature child:

> The advice I would give them to, the one I had, the one I have inside, that is don't get high, don't get up high about little things, don't be annoyed about little things, don't let your path be blocked by little things, being called black. You are black. I know it's an insult but every insult is not too bad. Think of your family, and if you can, if you can,

can say well I'll let that go by. Cos if you are little, you had a baby, literally a little child in your arms and it trying to get you hard and it hit you in the face and it break your glasses and a piece cut your face, you're not going to slap that little child. I don't tell you if, that someone outside did it, that you're going to knock their head off, but if you can just bear it, the little words, then that shouldn't so badly. Just don't take it on board. Find some sort of thing inside of YOU, to repel it and live long, live ha' more contented and everything there is open to you. (Respondent A)

The other example concerns treating others as you would be treated yourself. One respondent uses the metaphor of a mirror, of being a mirror-in-the-world, with oneself judged by one's own actions.

And the world see you as a mirror . . . because you are wondering how they are going to react to you. At the same time they too are wondering, wonder how that person's going to feel coming into our environment, coming into our home. And it what, what you reflect in that mirror, is what you are going to get out of it. And I try to teach my children in that way. And the same for every young people, if you want something, go out for it. Don't think that because you are of a different origin or a different skin colour that's going to prevent you. Yes, not everybody's going to open their door to you, but don't let it be a put off. Try another area. And I think that that's the advice I would be to any young people. If you have an ability and you know that there are certain demands that are required of you; certain expectations to be properly educated to meet the changing situation today. (Respondent D)

The sustenance for this moral framework seems to derive from a variety of sources, including the Christian church, family values taught in the Caribbean, external bureaucratic validation of achievement (examinations, qualifications), personal character, professional code of conduct and the supportive behaviour of, according to different individual accounts, either the majority or a minority of white peoples encountered.

However, the respondents do not regard their life histories as a complete triumph. Most feel that they could and should have achieved more. What they find especially hurtful is the way in which, when white people are asked to confront racism, their first reaction is to claim that white people are also discriminated against by minority ethnic groups.

I just have this ache because I can't understand why people find it so difficult, when black people say they've had a hard time. (Respondent H)

In summary, the moral resistance of our respondents to racisms has three dimensions: confronting and naming experiences as racisms, contrasting the brutalities of some white people with the cultured image of white people they had carried with them from the Caribbean, and constructing moral accounts of the type we have described.

Conclusion

In this chapter we have argued that a traditional view of professions as autonomous practitioners, operating from a perspective of improving public welfare, has been subjected to serious criticism. There are those who would argue that being a profession has a variety of implications, many of which are not desirable ones (Salvage 1985). The literature on professionalism within sociology has made relatively little reference to issues of ethnicity. In the early twenty-first century we are seeing the health service once again resort to the recruitment of 'overseas' nurses to solve its labour shortage. This chapter has examined some of the experiences of Caribbean migrants who came to the UK to train or work as nurses in the postwar period and the way in which they have negotiated their working lives in this country.

In responding to racism in the NHS, the Caribbean nurses in our study developed three strategies. First, they refused to assume that all negative experiences were attributable to racism. As Hall (1992) suggests, these respondents have other identities to draw upon which include student nurse status, age, gender and professional nurse status which cut across their experiences of racism and the processes of ethnic identity formation and which provide alternative structures within which to situate their experiences. Second, they have to learn to deal gradually and tentatively with what Porter (1993) describes as backstage racisms. Third, some experiences are construed both then and now as racisms and a sense of moral resistance is constructed.

The moral resistance may itself be thought of in three parts. First, the Caribbean nurses are confronted with experiences they name as racisms which, second, are in contrast to their socially learned predisposition to conceive of white peoples as cultured. The contrast is used as the opposition, out of which, third, are constructed accounts in which surviving challenging experiences confirms their own sense of moral worth. In surviving they have made considerable occupational contributions to British nursing.

We would like to thank our respondents and record our enormous respect and gratitude for their contributions to the NHS in the face of adversity. The research was funded by the Faculty of Health and Community Studies at De Montfort University, Leicester.

References

Acheson D (1998) *Independent Enquiry into Inequalities in Health*. The Stationery Office, London.

Adebimpe V R (1994) Race, Racism, and Epidemiological Surveys. *Hospital and Community Psychiatry* **45**(1): 27–31.

Adelstein A, Marmot M, Dean M G and Bradshaw S (1986) Comparison of mortality of Irish immigrants in England and Wales with that of Irish and British nationals. *Irish Medical Journal* **79**(7): 185–9.

Afshar H (1989) Gender roles and the 'moral economy of kin' among Pakistani women in West Yorkshire. *New Community* **15**(2): 211–25.

Ahmad W I U (1992) *The politics of 'race' and health*. The Race Relations Research Unit, University of Bradford and Bradford and Ilkely Community College, Bradford.

Ahmad W I U (ed) (1993) *'Race' and Health in Contemporary Britain*. Open University Press, Buckingham.

Ahmad W I U (1994) Reflections on consanguinity and the birth outcome debate. *Journal of Public Health Medicine* **16**(4): 423–38.

Ahmad W I U (1996a) The trouble with culture. In Kelleher D and Hillier S (eds) *Researching Cultural Differences in Health*. Routledge, London, pp. 190–219.

Ahmad W I U (1996b) Family obligations and social change among Asian communities. In Ahmad W I U and Atkin K (eds) *'Race' and Community Care*. Open University Press, Buckingham, pp. 52–72.

Ahmad W I U (1999) Ethnic statistics: better than nothing or worse than nothing? In Dorling D and Simpson S (eds) *Statistics in Society: the Arithmetic of Politics*. Arnold, London, pp. 124–31.

Ahmad W I U (ed) (2000) *Ethnicity, Disability and Chronic Illness*. Open University Press, Buckingham.

Ahmad W I U and Atkin K (eds) (1996) *'Race' and Community Care*. Open University Press, Buckingham.

Ahmad W I U, Atkin K and Chamba R (2000) Causing havoc among their children: parental and professional perspectives on consanguinity and childhood disability. In Ahmad W I U (ed) *Ethnicity, Disability and Chronic Illness*. Buckingham: Open University Press: 28–44.

Ahmad W I U, Kernohan E and Baker M (1989) Patient's choice of general practitioner: influence of patients' fluency in English and the ethnicity and sex of the doctor. *Journal of the Royal College of General Practitioners* **39**: 153–5.

Ahmad W, Baker M and Kernohan E (1991) General practitioners' perceptions of Asian and non-Asian patients. *Family Practice* **8**(1): 52–6.

Ahmad W I U and Sheldon T (1993) 'Race' and statistics. In Hammersley M (ed) *Social Research: Philosophy, Politics and Practice.* London, Sage, pp. 124–30.

Akinsanya J A (1988) Ethnic minority nurses, midwives and health visitors: what role for them in the National Health Service? *New Community* 14(3): 444–50.

Alladina S (1993) South Asian Languages in Britain. In Extra G and Vernhoeven L (eds) *Immigrant Languages in Europe.* Multilingual Matters, Clevedon.

Alleyne J, Papadoupoulos I and Tilki M (1994) Anti-Racism within transcultural education. *British Journal of Nursing* 3(12): 635–7.

Al-Rasheed M (1996) The Other-Others: hidden Arabs? In Peach C (ed) *Ethnicity in the 1991 Census Volume 2.* HMSO, London, pp. 206–20.

American Psychiatric Association (1995) *Diagnostic and Statistical Manual IV.* Washington DC.

American Speech-language Hearing Association Joint Subcommittee of the Executive Board on English Language Proficiency (1998) Students and professionals who speak English with accents and non-standard dialects: issues and recommendations. *Asha* 40 (supplement 18).

Amin K and Oppenheim C (1992) *Poverty in Black and White.* Child Poverty Action Group/Runnymede Trust, London.

Anderson D (1998) On being an advocate. *Registered Nurse* 61(9): 96.

Anderson J, Elfert H and Lai M (1989) Ideology and the clinical context: chronic illness, ethnicity and the discourse on normalisation. *Sociology of Health and Illness* 11(3): 253–78.

Andrews A and Jewson N (1993) Ethnicity and infant deaths: the implications of recent statistical evidence for materialist explanations. *Sociology of Health and Illness* 15(2): 137–56.

Andrews L B, Fullarton J E, Holtzman N A and Motulsky A G (eds) (1994) *Assessing Genetic Risks: Implications for Assessing Health and Social Policy.* Washington DC, National Academy Press.

Ang I (1996) The Curse of the Smile: Ambivalence and the 'Asian' Woman in Australian Multiculturalism. *Feminist Review* 52: 36–49.

Angastiniotis M, Kyriakidou S and Hadjiminas M (1986) How thalassaemia was controlled in Cyprus. *World Health Forum* 7: 291–7.

Anionwu E N (1991) Haemoglobinopathies (sickle cell disease and thalassaemia). *Words about action: review of services for black and minority ethnic people.* 4 National Association of Health Authorities and Trusts, Birmingham.

Anionwu E N (1993) Sickle cell and thalassaemia: community experiences and official response. In Ahmad W I U (ed) *'Race' and Health in Contemporary Britain.* Open University Press, Buckingham, pp. 76–95.

Anionwu E N (1996) Ethnic origin of sickle and thalassaemia counsellors: does it matter? In Kelleher D and Hillier S (eds) *Researching Cultural Differences in Health.* Routledge, London, pp. 160–89.

Anionwu E N, Patel N, Kanji G, Renges H and Brozovic M (1988) Counselling for prenatal diagnosis of sickle cell disease and beta-thalassaemia major: a four year experience. *Journal of Medical Genetics* **25**: 769–72.

Anonymous (1975) Language banks: put in interpreters, take out understanding. *Modern Health Care* **3**(2): 44–5.

Anonymous (1981) Study reveals multiple interpretations of phrases commonly used by doctors. *Connecticut Medicine* **45**(12): 799–800.

Anthias F (1998) Evaluating diaspora: beyond ethnicity? *Sociology* **32**(3): 557–80.

Anthias F and Yuval Davis N (1992) *Racialised Boundaries: Race, Gender, Colour and Class and the Anti-Racist Struggle.* Routledge, London.

Anwar M (1990) Ethnic classifications, ethnic monitoring and the 1991 Census. *New Community* **16**(4): 607–15.

Arai Y and Farrow S (1995) Access, expectations and communication: Japanese mothers' interactions with GPs in a pilot study in North London. *Public Health* **109**: 353–61.

Arber S (1990) Revealing women's health: reanalysing the General Household Survey. In Roberts H (ed) *Women's Health Counts.* Routledge, London, pp. 63–92.

Armstead C, Lawler K, Gorden G, Cross J and Gibbons J (1989) Relationship of racial stressors to blood pressure responses and anger expression in Black college students. *Health Psychology* **8**(5): 541–56.

Armstrong J (1982) *Nations Before Nationalism.* University of North Carolina Press, Chapel Hill.

Aspinall P (1995) Department of Health's requirement for mandatory collection of data on ethnic group of inpatients. *British Medical Journal* **311**: 1006–9.

Aspinall P (2000) The new 2001 census question set on cultural characteristics: is it useful for the monitoring of the health status of people from ethnic groups in Britain? *Ethnicity and Health* **5**(1): 33–40.

Atkin K (1996) An opportunity for change: voluntary sector provision in a mixed economy of care. In Ahmad W I U and Atkin K (eds) *'Race' and Community Care.* Open University Press, Buckingham, pp. 144–60.

Atkin K and Ahmad W I U (1996) Ethnicity and caring for a disabled child: the case of sickle cell or thalassaemia. *British Journal of Social Work* **26**: 755–75.

Atkin K, Ahmad W I U and Anionwu E N (1998) Screening and counselling for sickle cell disorders and thalassaemia: the experience of parents and health professionals. *Social Science and Medicine* **47**(11): 1639–51.

Atkin K and Rollings J (1996) Looking after their own? Family caregiving among Asian and Afro-Caribbean communities. In Ahmad W I U and Atkin K (eds) *'Race' and Community Care.* Open University Press, Buckingham, pp. 73–86.

Audit Commission (1994a) *Finding a Place: A Review of Mental Health Services for Adults.* HMSO, London.

Audit Commission (1994b) *What Seems To Be The Matter: Communication Between Hospitals and Patients.* HMSO, London.

Auerback M L (1995) Language Barriers in Medicine. *Journal of the American Medical Association* **274**(9): 683.

Bagley C (1971) The social aetiology of schizophrenia in immigrant groups. *International Journal of Social Psychiatry* **17**: 292–304.

Bahl M V (1987) *Asian mother and baby campaign: a report by the director Miss Veena Bahl.* Department of Health and Social Security, London.

Bailey-Holgate G (1996) Educating young adults about sickle cell and thalassaemia. *Health Visitor* **69**(12): 499–500.

Bains B and Chapman C (1996) Current practice in ante-natal screening for haemoglobin disorders in the UK. Paper presented to the UK Forum on Haemoglobin Disorders, 10 October 1996. Postgraduate Health Sciences Centre, Manchester.

Baker D W, Hayes R and Fortier J P (1998) Interpreter use and satisfaction with interpersonal aspects of care for Spanish-speaking patients. *Medical Care* **36**(10): 1461–70.

Bal P and Bal G (1995) *Health Care Needs of a Multi-Racial Society: A Practical Guide for Health Professionals.* Hawkar Publications, London.

Balarajan R and Bulusu L (1990) Mortality among immigrants in England and Wales, 1979–83. In Britton M (ed) *Mortality and Geography: A Review in the Mid-1980s.* OPCS (Series DS No. 9), London, pp. 103–21.

Balarajan R and Raleigh V S (1993) *Ethnicity and Health: a guide for the NHS.* Department of Health, London.

Balarajan R, Yuen P and Raleigh V S (1989) Ethnic differences in general practitioner consultations. *British Medical Journal* **229**: 958–60.

Banks M (1996) *Ethnicity: Anthropological Constructions.* Routledge, London.

Barclay L M, Sebastian E, Mills A E, Jones L K and Schmied V A (1993) A study of the services provided by the women's health nurses in a Sydney Area Health Service. *Australian Family Physician* **107**: 2016–19.

Barker C (1998) Cindy's a slut. *Sociology* **32**(1): 65–82.

Barker M (1981) *The New Racism.* Junction Books, London.

Barsky R F (1996) The interpreter as intercultural agent in convention refugee hearings. *The Translator* **2**(1): 45–63.

Barth F (ed) (1969) *Ethnic Groups and Boundaries: the Social Organisation of Culture Difference.* Allen & Unwin, London.

Bauman Z (1996) From pilgrim to tourist – or a short history of identity. In Hall S and du Gay P (eds) *Questions of Cultural Identity.* Sage Publications, London.

Baxter C (1988) *The Black Nurse: An Endangered Species.* Training in Health and Race, National Extension College, Cambridge.

Baxter C (1989) *Cancer Support and Ethnic Minority and Migrant Worker Communities.* CancerLink, London.

Baxter C (1998) Developing an agenda for promoting race equality in the nurse education curriculum. *NT Research* **3**(5): 339–48.

Baylav A (1996) Overcoming culture and language barriers. *The Practitioner* **240**: 403–6.

Becker H, Greer D, Hughes E and Strauss A (1961) *Boys in White*. University of Chicago Press, Chicago.

Beishon S, Modood T and Virdee S (1998) *Ethnic Minority Families*. Policy Studies Institute, London.

Beishon S, Virdee S and Hagell A (1995) *Nursing in a multi-ethnic NHS*. Policy Studies Institute, London.

Benzeval M and Judge K (1993) *The Development of Population-Based Need Indicators from Self-Reported Health Care Utilisation Data*. King's Fund Institute, London.

Benzeval M, Judge K and Solomon M (1992) *The Health Status of Londoners: A Comparative Perspective*. King's Fund, London.

Berthoud R and Beishon S (1997) People, families and households. In Modood T, Berthoud R, Lakey J, Nazroo J, Smith P, Virdee S and Beishon S (eds) *Ethnic Minorities in Britain: Diversity and Disadvantage*. Policy Studies Institute, London, pp. 18–59.

Bhopal R (undated) *Setting Priorities for Health Care for Ethnic Minority Groups*. Department of Epidemiology and Public Health, University of Newcastle upon Tyne.

Bhopal R (1988) Health care for Asians: conflict in need, demand and provision. In *Equity: a Pre-Requisite for Health*, Proceedings of the 1987 Summer Scientific Conference of the Faculty of Community Medicine.

Bhopal R and White M (1993) Health promotion for ethnic minorities: past, present and future. In Ahmad W I U (ed) *'Race' and Health in Contemporary Britain*. Open University Press, Buckingham.

Bhugra D and Bahl V (eds) (1999) *Ethnicity: An Agenda for Mental Health*. Gaskell, London.

Bhugra D, Hilwig M, Hossein B, Marceau H, Neehall J, Leff J, Mallett R and Der G (1996) First-contact incidence rates of schizophrenia in Trinidad and one-year follow-up. *British Journal of Psychiatry* **169**: 587–92.

Bhugra D, Leff J, Mallett R, Der G, Corridan B and Rudge S (1997) Incidence and outcome of schizophrenia in whites, African-Caribbeans and Asians in London. *Psychological Medicine* **27**: 791–8.

Blakemore K (1982) Health and illness among the elderly minority ethnic groups living in Birmingham: some new findings. *Health Trends* **14**: 69–73.

Blane D, Power C and Bartley M (1996) Illness Behaviour and the Measurement of Class Differentials in Morbidity. *Journal of the Royal Statistical Society* **156**(1): 77–92.

Boneham M (1989) Ageing and ethnicity in Britain: the case of elderly Sikh women in a Midlands town. *New Community* **15**(3): 447–59.

Bonnett A (1996) Anti-racism and the critique of 'white' identities. *New Community* **22**(1): 97–110.

Bourdieu P (1993) *The Field of Cultural Production*. Polity Press, London.

Bowes A and Domokos T M (1996) Pakistani women and maternity care: raising muted voices. *Sociology of Health and Illness* 18(1): 45–65.

Bowler I (1993a) 'They're not the same as us': midwives' stereotypes of South Asian descent maternity patients. *Sociology of Health and Illness* 15(2): 157–78.

Bowler I (1993b) Stereotypes of women of Asian descent in midwifery: some evidence. *Midwifery* 9: 7–16.

Bradby H (1995) Ethnicity and health: not a Black and White issue. *Sociology of Health and Illness* 17(3): 405–17.

Bradby H (1996) Genetics and racism. In Marteau T and Richards M (eds) *The Troubled Helix: Social and Psychological Implications of the New Human Genetics*. Cambridge University Press, Cambridge, pp. 295–316.

Brafman A (1995) Beware of the distorting interpreter. *British Medical Journal* 311: 1439.

Brenner P (1997) Issues of access in a diverse society. *The Hospice Journal* 12(2): 9–16.

Bromley Y (ed) (1974) *Soviet Ethnology and Anthropology Today*. Mouton, The Hague.

Bromley Y (1989) The theory of ethnos and ethnic processes in *Soviet Social Science. Comparative Studies in Society and Social Science* 31(3): 425–38.

Brown C (1984) *Black and White Britain*. Policy Studies Institute, London.

Brown D, Gary L, Greene A and Milburn N (1992) Patterns of social affiliation as predictors of depressive symptoms among urban Blacks. *Journal of Health and Social Behaviour* 33: 242–53.

Brozovic M and Anionwu E (1984) Sickle cell disease in Britain. *Journal of Clinical Pathology* 37: 1321–6.

Brozovic M, Davies S and Brownwell A (1987) Acute admissions of patients with sickle cell disease who live in Britain. *British Medical Journal* 294: 1206–8.

Bruni N (1988) A critical analysis of transcultural theory. *Australian Journal of Advanced Nursing* 15: 26–36.

Buchan J (1998) Your Country Needs You. *Health Service Journal* 108(5613): 22–5.

Bulmer M (1996) The ethnic group question in the 1991 Census of population. In Coleman D and Salt J (eds) *Ethnicity in the 1991 Census Volume 1*. HMSO, London: pp. 33–62.

Burr J A and Chapman T (1998) Some reflections on cultural and social considerations in mental health nursing. *Journal of Psychiatric and Mental Health Nursing* 5: 431–7.

Cameron E, Evers H, Badger F and Atkin K (1988) *District Nursing, the Disabled and the Elderly: Where are the Black Patients?* Community Care Project Working Paper No. 6, University of Birmingham.

Carlisle D (1996) A Nurse in Any Language. *Nursing Times* **92**(39): 26–7.

Cave A, Maharaj U, Gibson N and Jackson E (1995) Physician and immigrant patients. Cross cultural communication. *Canadian Family Physician* **41**(Oct): 1685–90.

Cesarani D (1996) The changing character of citizenship and nationality in Britain. In Cesarani D and Fulbrook M (eds) *Citizenship, Nationality and Migration in Europe*. Routledge, London, pp. 57–73.

Chan C (2000) A study of health services for the Chinese minority in Manchester. *British Journal of Nursing* **5**(3): 140–7.

Chapman T W (1995) Language barriers in Medicine. *Journal of the American Medical Association* **274**(9): 683–4.

Chapple A (1998) Iron deficiency anaemia in women of South Asian descent: a qualitative study. *Ethnicity and Health* **3**(3): 199–212.

Chevannes M (1989) Child rearing among Jamaican Families in Britain. *Health Visitor* **62**(2): 48–51.

Chevannes M (1995) Promoting multicultural care – nurses, children and their families. In Fatchett A (ed) *Caring for Health: From Childhood to Adolescence*. Baillere Tindall, London, pp. 93–122.

Chevannes M (1997) Nurses caring for families – issues in a multi-racial society. *Journal of Clinical Nursing* **6**: 161–7.

Chiu L F, Heywood P, Jordan J, McKinney P and Dowell T (1999) Balancing the equation: the significance of professional and lay perceptions in the promotion of cervical screening amongst minority ethnic women. *Critical Public Health* **9**(1): 5–21.

Chiu S (1989) Chinese elderly people: no longer a treasure at home. *Social Work Today* **10** August: 15–17.

Chriost D M G and Aitchison J (1998) Ethnic identities and language in Northern Ireland. *Area* **30**(4): 301–9.

Clark D (1994) At the crossroads: which direction for the hospices? (editorial). *Palliative Medicine* **8**(1): 1–3.

Clarke A (1991) Is non-directive genetic counselling possible? *Lancet* **338**: 998–1001.

Clarke A, Wallgren-Petterson C and Hughes H E (1992) Children with genetic diseases: who should pay? *Lancet* **339**: 1614–15.

Cochrane R and Bal S (1989) Mental hospital admission rates of immigrants to England: a comparison of 1971 and 1981. *Social Psychiatry and Psychiatric Epidemiology* **24**: 2–11.

Cochrane R and Stopes-Roe M (1981) Psychological symptom levels in Indian immigrants to England – a comparison with native English. *Psychological Medicine* **11**: 319–27.

Cohen A (1974) *Urban Ethnicity*. Tavistock, London.

Cohen A (1985) *The Symbolic Construction of Community*. Routledge, London.

Cohen R (1979) *Global Diasporas: An Introduction*. UCL Press, London.

Cole E, Leavey G, King M, Johnson-Sabine E and Hoar A (1995) Pathways to care for patients with a first episode of psychosis: a comparison of ethnic groups. *British Journal of Psychiatry* **167**: 770–76.

Coleman D and Salt J (eds) (1996a) *Ethnicity in the 1991 Census Volume 1.* HMSO, London, pp. 33–62.

Coleman D and Salt J (1996b) The ethnic group question in the 1991 Census: a new landmark in British social statistics. In Coleman D and Salt J (eds) (1996a) *Ethnicity in the 1991 Census Volume 1.* HMSO, London, pp. 1–32.

Commander M J, Dharan S P, Odell S M and Surtees P G (1997) Access to mental health care in an inner city health district II: association with demographic factors. *British Journal of Psychiatry* **170**: 317–20.

Commission for Racial Equality (1983) *Ethnic Minority Hospital Staff.* Commission for Racial Equality, London.

Commission for Racial Equality (1992) *Race Relations Code of Practice for Primary Health Care Services.* Commission for Racial Equality, London.

Connelly N (1988) *Ethnic Record Keeping and Monitoring in Service Delivery.* Policy Studies Institute, London.

Coronary Prevention Group (1986) *Coronary Heart Disease and Asians in Britain.* CPG/Confederation of Indian Organizations, London.

Court S D M (1976) *Fit for the Future: Report of the Committee on Child Health Services.* Cmnd 6684. London: HMSO.

Cox O C (1948) *Caste, Class and Race.* Monthly Review Press, New York.

Culley L A (1996) A critique of multiculturalism in health care: the challenge for nurse education. *Journal of Advanced Nursing* **23**: 564–70.

Culley L A (1997) Ethnicity, health and sociology in the nursing curriculum. *Social Sciences in Health* **3**(1): 28–40.

Culley L (2000) Working with diversity: beyond the factfile. In Davies C, Finlay L and Bullman A (eds) *Changing Practice in Health and Social Care.* Sage/Open University Press, London, pp. 131–42.

Currer C (1986) Concepts of mental well- and ill-being: the case of Pathan mothers in Britain. In Currer C and Stacey M (eds) *Concepts of Health and Illness.* Berg, Leamington Spa, pp. 181–314.

Daniel W W (1968) *Racial Discrimination in England.* Penguin, Harmondsworth.

Davidson M J (1997) *The Black and Ethnic Minority Worker: Cracking the Concrete Ceiling.* Paul Chapman Publishing, London.

Davies C (1995) *Gender and the Professional Predicament in Nursing.* Open University Press, Buckingham.

Davies S (1993) Services for people with haemoglobinopathy. *British Medical Journal* **308**: 1051–2.

Davies S, Cronin E, Gill M, Greengross P, Hickman M and Normand C (2000) Screening for sickle cell disease and thalassaemia systematic review with supplementary research. *Health Technology Assessment* **4**(3).

Davies S C, Modell B and Wonke B (1993) The haemoglobinopathies: impact upon black and ethnic minority people. In Hopkins A and Bahl

V (eds) *Access to health care for people from black and ethnic minorities.* Royal College of Physicians, London, pp. 147–68.

Davies S, Thornicroft G, Leese M, Higgingbotham A and Phelan M (1996) Ethnic differences in risk of compulsory psychiatric admission among representative cases of psychosis in London. *British Medical Journal* **312**: 533–7.

Davis D L (1984) Medical misinformation: communication between Outport Newfoundland women and their physicians. *Social Science and Medicine* **18**(3): 273–8.

Day M (1994) Racial discrimination: professional implications. *Journal of Interprofessional Care* **8**(2): 135–40.

Dein S (1997) ABC of mental health: mental health in a multi-ethnic society. *British Medical Journal* **315**: 473–6.

DeLamater J (1982) Response-effects of question content. In Dijkstra W and Van der Zouwen J (eds) *Response Behaviour in the Survey-Interview.* Academic Press, London, pp. 13–48.

Department of Health (1990a) *National Health Service and Community Care Act.* HMSO, London.

Department of Health (1990b) *Community Care in the Next Decade and Beyond. Policy Guidance.* HMSO, London.

Department of Health (1991) *The Patient's Charter: Raising the Standard.* HMSO, London.

Department of Health (1993a) *Report of a Standing Medical Advisory Committee on Sickle Cell, Thalassaemia and Other Haemoglobinopathies.* HMSO, London.

Department of Health (1993b) *The Health of the Nation Key Areas Handbook: HIV/AIDS and Sexual Health.* HMSO, London.

Department of Health (1993c) *Ethnicity and Health: A Guide for the NHS.* Department of Health, London.

Department of Health (1996) *Directory of Ethnic Minority Initiatives.* Department of Health, London.

Department of Health (1997) *The New NHS: modern, dependable.* The Stationery Office, London.

Department of Health (1998a) *Working Together: Securing a quality workforce for the NHS.* Department of Health, London.

Department of Health (1998b) *Tackling Racial Harassment in the NHS. A Plan for Action.* Department of Health, London.

Department of Health (1998c) *They look after their own, don't they? Inspection of Community Care Services for Black and Ethnic Minority Older People.* Social Care Group, Social Services Inspectorate, London.

Department of Health (1998d) *Our Healthier Nation.* The Stationery Office, London.

Department of Health (1999) *Saving Lives. Our Healthier Nation.* Cm 4386. The Stationery Office, London.

Department of Health (2000) *The Vital Connection: An Equalities Framework for the NHS.* Department of Health, London.

De Santis L (1994) Making anthropology clinically relevant to nursing care. *Journal of Advanced Nursing* **20**: 707–15.

Diaz-Duque O (1982) Advice from an interpreter. *American Journal of Nursing.* September 1982: 1380–82.

Dickens L (1994) Wasted Resources? Equal Opportunities in Employment. In Sisson K (ed) *Personnel Management.* Blackwell, Oxford, pp. 253–96.

Directive 95/46/EC of the European Parliament and Council – 24 October 1995: On the protection of individuals with regard to the processing of personal data and the free movement of such data. *Official Journal of the European Communities* (OJ) L 281/31, **38**, 23 November 1995.

Dodd W (1983) Do interpreters affect consultations? *Family Practice* **1**(1): 42–7.

Donaldson L (1986) Health and social status of elderly Asians: a community survey. *British Medical Journal* **293**: 1079–82.

Donovan J (1984) Ethnicity and health: a research review. *Social Science and Medicine* **19**(7): 663–70.

Douglas J (1995) Developing anti-racist health promotion strategies. In Bunton R, Nettleton S and Burrows R (eds) *The Sociology of Health Promotion.* Routledge, London, pp. 70–77.

Doyal L, Gee F, Hunt G, Mellor J and Pennell I (1980) *Migrant Workers in the National Health Service: Report on a Preliminary Survey.* Social Science Research Council, London.

Draper E (1991) *Risky business: genetic testing and exclusionary practices in the hazardous workplace.* Cambridge University Press, Cambridge.

Drennan G (1996) Counting the cost of language services in psychiatry. *South African Medical Journal* **86**(4): 343–5.

Dressler W (1988) Social consistency and psychological distress. *Journal of Health and Social Behaviour* **29**: 79–91.

Dressler W (1993) Type A behavior: contextual effects within a southern Black community. *Social Science and Medicine* **36**(3): 289–95.

Durham M (1991) *Sex and Politics – The Family and Morality in the Thatcher Years.* Macmillan, London.

Dyson S (1999) Genetic screening and ethnic minorities. *Critical Social Policy* **19**(2): 195–215.

Dyson S, Davis V and Rahman R (1993) Thalassaemia: current community knowledge in Manchester. *Health Visitor* **66**(12): 447–8.

Dyson S, Fielder A and Kirkham M (1996a) Midwives' and senior student midwives' knowledge of haemoglobinopathies in England. *Midwifery* **12**: 23–30.

Dyson S, Fielder A and Kirkham M (1996b) The educational implications of a study of midwives' and senior student midwives' knowledge concerning haemoglobinopathies. *Modern Midwife* **6**(7): 22–5.

Dyson S, Fielder A and Kirkham M (1996c) Haemoglobinopathies, antenatal screening and the midwife. *British Journal of Midwifery* **4**(6): 319–22.

Eade J (1995) The power of the experts: the plurality of beliefs and practices concerning health and illness among Bangladeshis. Unpublished manuscript. Roehampton Institute, London.

Ebden P, Bhatt A, Carey O J and Harrison B (1988) The bilingual consultation. *Lancet* 1(8581): 347.

Ellis B (1990) *Racial Equality: The Nursing Profession*. King's Fund Equal Opportunities Task Force, King's Fund, London.

Esmail A and Everington S (1993) Racial discrimination against doctors from ethnic minorities. *British Medical Journal* **306**: 691–2.

Esmail A, Nelson P, Primarolo D and Toma T (1995) Acceptance into medical school and racial discrimination. *British Medical Journal* **310**: 501–2.

Esmail A, Everington S and Doyle H (1998) Racial discrimination in the allocation of distinction awards? Analysis of list of award holders by type of award, speciality and region. *British Medical Journal* **316**: 193–5.

Etzioni A (1969) *The Semi-Professions and their Organization*. Free Press, New York.

European Parliament and Council Directive 95/46/EC, 24 October 1995: On the protection of individuals with regard to the processing of personal data and the free movement of such data. *Official Journal of the European Communities* (OJ) L 281/31, **38**, 23 November 1995.

Farrar M (1999) *Primary Care Trusts: Establishing Better Services*. NHS Executive, Leeds.

Fenton S (1988) Health work and growing old: the Afro-Caribbean experience. *New Community* 14(3): 426–43.

Fenton S (1999) *Ethnicity. Racism, Class and Culture*. Macmillan, Basingstoke.

Fenton S, Hughes A and Hine C (1995) Self-assessed health, economic status and ethnic origin. *New Community* 21(1): 55–68.

Fenton S and Sadiq-Sangster A (1996) Culture, relativism and the expression of mental distress: South Asian women in Britain. *Sociology of Health and Illness* 18(1): 66–85.

Fernando S (1991) *Mental Health, Race and Culture*. Macmillan, Basingstoke.

Field D (1989) *Nursing the Dying*. Routledge, London

Field D, Hockey J and Small N (1997) *Death, Gender and Ethnicity*. Routledge, London.

Fitzgerald M and Sibbitt R (1997) *Ethnic Monitoring in Police Forces: a Beginning*. Home Office Research Study 173, London.

Fleming A (1982) *Sickle Cell Disease: a Handbook for the General Clinician*. Churchill Livingstone, London.

Frankenberg R (1993) *White Women, Race Matters – The Social Construction of Whiteness*. Routledge, London.

Frankenburg W and Dodds J (1967) The Denver development screening. *The Journal of Paediatrics* 71(2): 181–91.

Franklin I (1988) Services for sickle cell disease: unified approach needed. *British Medical Journal* **296** (27 February 1988): 592.

Freedman J and Coombs G (1996) *Narrative Therapy: the Social Construction of Preferred Realities*. W W Norton, New York.

Freidson E (1970) *Professional Dominance: the Social Structure of Medical Care.* Atherton Press, New York.

Fryer P (1984) *Staying Power: The History of Black People in Britain.* Pluto Press, London.

Gabe J, Kelleher D and Williams G (eds) (1994) *Challenging Medicine.* Routledge, London.

Gabe J and Thorogood N (1986) Prescribed drug use and the management of everyday life: the experience of black and white working-class women. *Sociological Review* **34**(4): 737–72.

Gabriel J and Ben-Tovim G (1978) Marxism and the concept of racism. *Economy and Society* 7(2): 118–54.

George M (1994) Racism in nursing. *Nursing Standard* **8**(18): 20–1.

Gerrish K (1997) Preparation of nurses to meet the needs of an ethnically diverse society: educational implications. *Nurse Education Today* **17**(5): 359–65.

Gerrish K (1999) Inequalities in service provision: an examination of institutional influences on the provision of district nursing care to minority ethnic communities. *Journal of Advanced Nursing* **30**(6): 1263–71.

Gerrish K, Husband C and Mackenzie J (1996) *Nursing for a Multi-Ethnic Society.* Open University Press, Buckingham.

Gilliam S J, Jarman B, White P and Law R (1989) Ethnic differences in consultation rates in urban general practice. *British Medical Journal* **299**: 953–7.

Gilroy P (1987) *There Ain't No Black in the Union Jack.* Hutchinson, London.

Gilroy P (1993) *The Black Atlantic.* Verso, London.

Gilroy P (1997) Diaspora and the detours of identity. In Woodward K (ed) *Identity and Difference.* Sage, London, pp. 299–346.

Glass R (1960) *The Newcomers.* Allen & Unwin, London.

Glickman M (1997) *Making Palliative Care Better: Quality Improvement, Multi-Professional Audit and Standards.* Occasional Paper 12. National Council for Hospice and Specialist Palliative Care Services, London.

Godlee F (1996) The GMC, racism and complaints against doctors. *British Medical Journal* **312**: 1314–15.

Goldberg D (1993) *Racist Culture: Philosophy and the Politics of Meaning.* Blackwell, Oxford.

Goode W (1960) Encroachment, charlatanism and the emerging profession: psychology, sociology and medicine. *American Sociological Review* **25**: 902–14.

Gordon P and Newnham A (1985) *Passport to Benefits? Racism in Social Security.* Child Poverty Action Group/Runnymede Trust, London.

Graham H (1992) Budgeting for health: mothers in low-income households. In Glendinning C and Millar J (eds) *Women and Poverty in Britain the 1990s.* Harvester Wheatsheaf, Hemel Hempstead.

Green J (1989) *Death with Dignity: Meeting the Spiritual Needs of Patients in a Multi-Cultural Society.* Macmillan Magazines, London.

Green J (1992) *Death with Dignity: Meeting the Spiritual Needs of Patients in a Multi-Cultural Society* (Vol. Two). Macmillan Magazines, London.

Greenslade L, Madden M and Pearson M (1997) From visible to invisible: the 'problem' of the health of Irish people in Britain. In Marks L and Worboys M (eds) *Migrants, Minorities and Health.* Routledge, London, pp. 147–78.

Griffiths R (1960) (Reprinted 1986) *The Abilities of Babies.* The Test Agency, High Wycombe.

Grillo R (1989) *Dominant Languages: language and hierarchy in Britain and France.* Cambridge University Press, Cambridge.

Gunaratnam Y (1993) *Checklist Health and Race: A Starting Point for Managers on Improving Services for Black Populations.* King's Fund, London.

Gunaratnam Y (1997) Culture is not enough: a critique of multi-culturalism in palliative care. In Field D, Hockey J and Small N (eds) *Death, Gender and Ethnicity.* Routledge, London, pp. 166–86.

Gunaratnam Y, Bremner I, Pollock L and Weir C (1998) Anti-discrimination, emotions and professional practice. *European Journal of Palliative Care* 5(4): 122–4

Haffner L (1992) Translation is not enough – interpreting in a medical setting. *West Journal of Medicine* 157: 255–9.

Hagenaars J and Heinen T (1982) Effects of role independent characteristics on responses. In Dijkstra W and Van der Zouwen J (eds) *Response Behaviour in the Survey-Interview.* Academic Press, London, pp. 91–130.

Hall D M (1996) (ed) (3rd edn) *Health for All Children.* Oxford University Press, Oxford.

Hall S (1990) Cultural identity and diaspora. In Rutherford J (ed) *Identity: Community, Culture, Difference.* Lawrence & Wishart, London, pp. 222–37.

Hall S (1992) The new ethnicities. In Donald J and Rattansi A (eds) *'Race', Culture and Difference.* London, Sage, pp. 252–9.

Hall S (1996a) New ethnicities. In Morley D and Kuan-Hsing C (eds) *Stuart Hall – Critical Dialogues in Cultural Studies.* Routledge, London, pp. 441–9.

Hall S (1996b) Who needs identity? In Hall S and du Gay P (eds) *Questions of Cultural Identity.* Sage, London, pp. 1–17.

Handy S, Chithiramohan R N, Ballard C G and Silveira W R (1991) Ethnic differences in adolescent self-poisoning: a comparison of Asian and Caucasian groups. *Journal of Adolescence* 14: 157–62.

Harding S and Maxwell R (1997) Differences in mortality of migrants. In Drever F and Whitehead M (eds) *Health Inequalities.* Office for National Statistics, London, pp. 108–21.

Harper P (1992) Genetics and public health. *British Medical Journal* 304: 721.

Harris C (1993) Post-war migration and the industrial reserve army. In James W and Harris C (eds) *Inside Babylon: the Caribbean Diaspora in Britain*. Verso, London, pp. 9–54.

Harrison G, Holton A, Neilson D, Owens D, Boot D and Cooper J (1989) Severe mental disorder in Afro-Caribbean patients: some social, demographic and service factors. *Psychological Medicine* **19**: 683–96.

Harrison G, Owens D, Holton A, Neilson D and Boot D (1988) A prospective study of severe mental disorder in Afro-Caribbean patients. *Psychological Medicine* **18**: 643–57.

Hartrick G (1994) Family nursing assessment: meeting the challenge of health promotion. *Journal of Advanced Nursing* **20**(7): 85–91.

Hatton D C and Webb T (1993) Information transmission in bilingual, bicultural contexts: a field study of community health nurses and interpreters. *Journal of Community Health Nursing* **10**(3): 137–47.

Hayes L (1995) Unequal access to midwifery care: a continuing problem? *Journal of Advanced Nursing* **21**: 702–7.

Health Education Authority (1994) *Health-Related Resources for Black and Minority Ethnic Groups*. Health Education Authority, London.

Healy P (1996) Equality Matters. *Nursing Standard* **10**(29): 22–3.

Hek G (1991) Contact with Asian elders. *Journal of District Nursing* 13–15 December.

Henley A (1983) *Asians in Britain. Caring for Hindus and their Families: Religious Aspects of Care*. National Extension College, Cambridge.

Henley A (1991) *Caring for Everyone*. National Extension College, Cambridge.

Hickling F W (1991) Psychiatric hospital admission rates in Jamaica. *British Journal of Psychiatry* **159**: 817–21.

Hickling F W and Rodgers-Johnson P (1995) The incidence of first contact schizophrenia in Jamaica. *British Journal of Psychiatry* **167**: 193–6.

Hicks C (1982) Racism in nursing. *Nursing Times* 5 May 1982 and 12 May 1982.

Hill D and Penso D (1995) *Opening Doors: Improving Access to Hospice and Specialist Care Services by Members of Black and Ethnic Minority Communities*. National Council of Hospice and Specialist Palliative Care Services, London.

Hill S A (1994) *Sickle Cell Disease in Low Income Families*. Temple University Press, Philadephia.

Hill-Collins P (1991) *Black Feminist Thought – Knowledge, Consciousness, and the Politics of Empowerment*. Routledge, London.

Hilton C (1996) Collecting ethnic group data for in-patients: is it useful? *British Medical Journal* **313**: 923–5.

Hobbs P, McGuinness H and Lambert C (1989) Breast screening: meeting the language needs of ethnic minorities. *Journal of the Institute of Health Education* **27**(3): 157–61.

Hogg C and Modell B (1998) *Sickle Cell and Thalassaemia: Achieving Health Gain*. Health Education Authority, London.

Holmes C (1990) Alternatives to natural science foundations for nursing. *International Journal of Nursing Studies* 27(3): 187–97.

Holmes P (1990) Telephone translators. *Nursing Times* 86(28): 22–3.

hooks b (1989) *Talking Back*. Sheba Feminist Publishers, London.

Hornberger J C, Gibson C D, Wood W, Dequeldre C, Corso I, Palla B and Bloch D (1996) Eliminating language barriers for non-English-speaking patients. *Medical Care* 34(8): 845–56.

Hornberger J, Itakura H and Wilson S R (1997) Bridging language and cultural barriers between physician and patients. *Public Health Reports* 112(Sept./Oct.): 410–17.

Hughes A O, Fenton S and Hine C E (1996) Strategies for sampling black and ethnic minority populations. *Journal of Public Health Medicine* 17(2): 187–92.

Hurstfield J (1998) *Equal Opportunities and Monitoring in NHS Trusts*. NHS Equal Opportunities Unit, NHS Executive, Department of Health.

Hyman H (1954) *Interviewing in Social Research*. University of Chicago Press, Chicago.

Iganski P, Mason D, Humphreys A and Watkins M (1998) The 'Black nurse': ever an endangered species? *NT Research* 3(5): 325–38.

Jackson C (1990) Controversy surrounds new 'language line'. *Health Visitor* 63(9): 294.

Jadhav S (1996) The cultural origins of Western depression. *International Journal of Social Psychiatry* 42(4): 269–86.

Jamdagni L (1996) *Purchasing for Black Populations*. King's Fund, London.

James W (1993) Migration, racism and identity formation: the Caribbean experience in Britain. In James W and Harris C (eds) *Inside Babylon: the Caribbean Diaspora in Britain*. Verso, London, pp. 231–87.

James N and Field D (1992) The Routinization of Hospice: Charisma and Bureaucratization. *Social Science and Medicine* 34(12): 1362–75.

Jenkins R (1997) *Rethinking Ethnicity*. Sage, London.

Jenkins R and Solomos J (eds) (1989) *Racism and Equal Opportunity Policies in the 1980s*. Cambridge University Press, Cambridge.

Jewson N and Mason D (1986) The theory and practice of equal opportunity policies: liberal and radical. *Sociological Review* 34(2): 307–34.

Johnson M R D (1992) Health and social services. *New Community* 18(4): 611–18.

Johnson M R D and Gill P S (1995) Ethnic monitoring and equity: collecting data is just the beginning (editorial). *British Medical Journal* 310: 890.

Johnson T (1972) *Professions and Power*. Macmillan, London.

Jones S (1991) 'We are all cousins under the skin'. *The Independent* 12 December.

Jones D and Gill P (1998) Breaking down language barriers. *British Medical Journal* 316: 1476.

Kapasi R (1995) *Speaking Out: The Experiences of Black Elders with Strokes in Sandwell*. Sandwell Health Authority, Birmingham.

Karmi G (1992) *The Ethnic Factfile*. The Health and Ethnicity Programme, North East and North West Thames Regional Health Authorities, London.

Karmi G (1996) *The Ethnic Health Handbook. A Factfile for Health Care Professionals*. Blackwell Science, Oxford.

Karmi G, Abdulrahim D, Pierpoint T and McKeigue P (1994) *Suicide among Ethnic Minorities and Refugees in the UK*. North East and North West Thames Regional Health Authorities, London.

Karmi G and Horton C (1993) *Guidelines for the Implementation of Ethnic Monitoring in Health Service Provision*. North East and North West Thames Regional Health Authorities, London.

Kelleher D (1996) A defence of the use of the terms 'ethnicity' and 'culture'. In Kelleher D and Hillier S (eds) *Researching Cultural Differences in Health*. Routledge, London, pp. 69–90.

Kim Y (1992) Intercultural communication competence: a systems-theoretic view. In Gudykunst W B and Kim Y Y (eds) *Readings on Communication with Strangers*. McGraw-Hill, New York.

King D K (1988) Multiple jeopardy, multiple consciousness: the context of a black feminist ideology. *Signs* **14**(1): 42–72.

King M, Coker E, Leavey G, Hoare A and Johnson-Sabine E (1994) Incidence of psychotic illness in London: comparison of ethnic groups. *British Medical Journal* **309**: 1115–9.

King's Fund (1990) *Racial Equality: the Nursing Profession*. King's Fund Equal Opportunities Task Force, London.

King's Fund (1998) *London's Mental Health. The Report to the King's Fund London Commission*. King's Fund, London.

Kleinman A (1987) Anthropology and psychiatry: the role of culture in cross-cultural research on illness. *British Journal of Psychiatry* **151**: 447–54.

Krause I (1989) Sinking heart: a Punjabi communication of distress. *Social Science and Medicine* **29**(4): 563–75.

Krieger N (1990) Racial and gender discrimination: risk factors for high blood pressure? *Social Science and Medicine* **30**(12): 1273–81.

Lambert H and Sevak L (1996) Is 'cultural difference' a useful concept? Perceptions of health and the sources of ill health among Londoners of South Asian origin. In Kelleher D and Hillier S (eds) *Researching Cultural Differences*. Routledge, London, pp. 124–59.

Law I (1996) *Racism, Ethnicity and Social Policy*. Prentice-Hall, Hemel Hempstead.

Lawrence D (1974) *Black Migrants, White Natives*. Cambridge University Press, London.

Le Var R M H (1998) Improving educational preparation for transcultural health care. *Nurse Education Today* **18**(7): 519–33.

Lee E D, Rosenberg C R, Sixsmith D M, Pang D and Abularrage J (1998) Does a physician-patient language difference increase the probability of hospital admission? *Academic Emergency Medicine* **5**(1): 86–9.

Lee-Cunin M (1989) *Daughters of Seacole. A Study of Black Nurses in West Yorkshire.* West Yorkshire Low Pay Unit, Batley.

Leff J (1988) *Psychiatry around the globe: a transcultural view.* Gaskell, London.

Leininger M (1978) *Transcultural Nursing: Concepts, Theories and Practice.* John Wiley, New York.

Leininger M (ed) (1991) *Culture Care, Diversity and Universality: a Theory of Nursing.* National League for Nursing Press, New York.

Leman P (1997) Interpreter use in an inner city accident and emergency department. *Journal of Accident and Emergency Medicine* **14**(2): 98–100.

Levin J (1994) Religion and health: is there an association, is it valid and is it causal? *Social Science and Medicine* **38**(11): 1475–82.

Linguistic Minorities Project (1985) *The Other Languages of England.* Routledge, London.

Lipsedge M (1993) Mental health: access to care for black and ethnic minority people. In Hopkins A and Bahl V (eds) *Access to health care for people from black and ethnic minorities.* Royal College of Physicians, London.

Lister P (1999) A taxonomy for developing cultural competence. *Nurse Education Today* **19**: 313–18.

Littlewood R (1992) Psychiatric diagnosis and racial bias: empirical and interpretative approaches. *Social Science and Medicine* **34**(2): 141–9.

Littlewood R and Lipsedge M (1988) Psychiatric illness among British Afro-Caribbeans. *British Medical Journal* **296**: 950–51.

Lloyd K (1993) Depression and anxiety among Afro-Caribbean general practice attenders in Britain. *International Journal of Social Psychiatry* **39**: 1–9.

Lucas D and Ware H (1977) Language differences and the family planning survey. *Studies in Family Planning* **8**(9): 233–6.

Macpherson W (1999) *The Stephen Lawrence Inquiry: report of an inquiry by Sir William Macpherson.* (Cm 4262-I) Stationery Office, London.

Mallik M (1997a) Advocacy in nursing – a review of the literature. *Journal of Advanced Nursing* **25**: 130–38.

Mallik M (1997b) Advocacy in nursing – perceptions of practising nurses. *Journal of Clinical Nursing* **6**: 303–13.

Manton A (1998) Advocacy – an integral part of emergency nursing. *Journal of Emergency Nursing* **24**: 113–14.

Marmot M, Adelstein A and Bulusu L (1984) *Immigrant Mortality in England and Wales 1970–1978.* HMSO, London.

Martin G W (1998) Communication breakdown or ideal speech situation: the problem of nurse advocacy. *Nursing Ethics* **5**(2): 147–57.

Mason D (1995) *Race and Ethnicity in Modern Britain.* Oxford University Press, Oxford.

Mason E (1990) The Asian Mother and Baby Campaign (The Leicestershire Experience). *The Journal of the Royal Society of Health* **110**(1): 1–4, 9.

Maxwell R and Harding S (1998) Mortality of migrants from outside England and Wales by marital status. *Population Trends* **91**: 15–22.

Mayor V (1996) Investing in people: personal and professional development of black nurses. *Health Visitor* **69**(1): 20–3.

McAvoy B, Davis P, Raymont A and Gribben B (1994) The Waikato Medical Care Survey 1991–1992. *New Zealand Medical Journal* **107**: 388–433.

McCabe F and Rocheron Y (1985) Survey of health visiting in antenatal care. *British Medical Journal* **291**: 794–6.

McCormick A and Rosenbaum M (1990) *1981–1982 Morbidity Statistics from General Practice, Third National Study: Socio-Economic Analysis.* Series M85 No. 2, HMSO, London.

McGee P (1992) *Teaching Transcultural Care: A Guide for Teachers of Nursing and Health Care.* Chapman & Hall, London.

McGovern D and Cope R (1987) First psychiatric admission rates of first and second generation Afro-Caribbeans. *Social Psychiatry* **22**: 139–49.

McIvor R J (1994) Making the most of interpreters. *British Journal of Psychiatry* **165**(2): 268.

McKenzie K (1995) Racial Discrimination in Medicine. *British Medical Journal* **310**: 478–9.

McKenzie K and Crowcroft N S (1996) Describing race, ethnicity and culture in medical research. *British Medical Journal* **312**: 1054.

McKenzie K, van Os J, Fahy T, Jones P, Harvey I, Toone B and Murray R (1995) Psychosis with good prognosis in Afro-Caribbean people now living in the United Kingdom. *British Medical Journal* **311**: 1325–8.

McManus I C, Richards P, Winder B C, Sproston K A and Styles V (1995) Medical school applicants from ethnic minority groups: identifying if and when they are disadvantaged. *British Medical Journal* **310**: 496–502.

McNaught A (1987) *Health Action and Ethnic Minorities.* Bedford Square Press/NCHR, London.

Mellor P and Shilling C (1997) *Re-Forming The Body – Religion, Community and Modernity.* Sage, London.

Meltzer H, Gill B, Petticrew M and Hinds K (1995) *The Prevalence of Psychiatric Morbidity among Adults Living in Private Households.* HMSO, London.

Mensah J (1996) Everybody's problem. *Nursing Times* **92**(22): 26–7.

Mental Health Foundation (1995) *Mental Health in Black and Minority Ethnic People: The Fundamental Facts.* Mental Health Foundation, London.

Merrill J and Owens J (1986) Ethnic differences in self-poisoning: a comparison of Asian and White groups. *British Journal of Psychiatry* **148**: 708–12.

Merrill J, Owens J, Wynne S and Whittington R (1990) Asian suicides. *British Journal of Psychiatry* (letter) **156**: 748–9.

Meryn S (1998) Improving doctor-patient communication. *British Medical Journal* **316**: 1922–30.

Miers M (2000) *Gender Issues and Nursing Practice*. Macmillan Press – now Palgrave, Basingstoke.

Miles R (1982) *Racism and Migrant Labour*. Routledge and Kegan Paul, London.

Miles R (1989) *Racism*. Routledge, London.

Miles R (1993) *Racism after 'Race Relations'*. Routledge, London.

Miles R (1996) Racism and nationalism in the United Kingdom: a view from the periphery. In Barot R (ed) *The Racism Problematic: Contemporary Sociological Debates on Race and Ethnicity*. Edwin Mellen Press, Lewiston.

Mirza H S (1992) *Young Female and Black*. Routledge, London.

Mitchell P, Malak A and Small D (1998) Bilingual professionals in community mental health services. *Australian and New Zealand Journal of Psychiatry* **32**: 424–33.

Modell B and Anionwu E (1996) Guidelines for screening for haemoglobin disorders: service specifications for low- and high-prevalence district health authorities. In NHS Centre for Reviews and Dissemination *Ethnicity and Health: reviews of literature for purchasers in the areas of cardiovascular disease, mental health and haemoglobinopathies*. University of York, York, pp. 127–78.

Modell B, Kuliev A and Wagner M (1991) *Community Genetic Services in Europe*. WHO Regional Publications, European Series, No. 38. World Health Organization, Copenhagen.

Modell M and Modell B (1990) Genetic screening for ethnic minorities. *British Medical Journal* **300**: 1702–4.

Modell M, Wonke B, Khan M, See Tai S, Lloyd M and Modell B (1998) A multidisciplinary approach for improving services in primary care: randomised controlled trial of screening for haemoglobin disorders. *British Medical Journal* **317**(7161): 788–91.

Modood T (1990) Catching up with Jesse Jackson: being oppressed and being somebody. *New Community* 7(1): 85–96.

Modood T (1998) Anti-essentialism, multiculturalism and the 'recognition' of religious groups. *The Journal of Political Philosophy* 6(4): 378–99

Modood T, Beishon S and Virdee S (1994) *Changing Ethnic Identities*. Policy Studies Institute, London.

Modood T, Berthoud R, Lakey J, Nazroo J, Smith P, Virdee S and Beishon S (1997) *Ethnic Minorities in Britain: Diversity and Disadvantage*. Policy Studies Institute, London.

Moreton J and Macfarlane A (1991) (2nd edn) *Child Health and Surveillance*. Blackwell Scientific, Oxford.

MSF (1997) *The Tables Are Bare: a Briefing on the Continuing Inability of the NHS to Meet its own Equal Opportunities Goals in Respect of Ethnic Minority Staff*. Manufacturing, Science and Finance, London.

Mulholland J (1995) Nursing, humanism and transcultural theory: the bracketing out of reality. *Journal of Advanced Nursing* **22**: 442–9.

Munro R (1999) 'There's sin in them there genes'. *Nursing Times* **95**(33): 28–9.

Musser-Granski J and Carrillo D F (1997) The use of bilingual, bicultural paraprofessionals in mental health services: issues for hiring, training, and supervision. *Community Mental Health Journal* **33**(1): 51–60.

Naish J, Brown J and Denton B (1994) Intercultural consultations: investigation of factors that deter non-English speaking women from attending their general practitioners for cervical screening. *British Medical Journal* **309**: 1126–9.

Narayanasamy A (1999) Transcultural mental health nursing 1: benefits and limitations *British Journal of Nursing* **8**(10): 664–8.

National Association of Health Authorities and Trusts (1989) *Action Not Words: A Strategy to Improve Health Services for Black and Minority Ethnic Groups*. National Association of Health Authorities and Trusts, Birmingham.

National Council for Hospice and Specialist Palliative Care Services (1995) *Specialist Palliative Care: A Statement of Definitions*. Occasional Paper 8. National Council for Hospice and Specialist Palliative Care Services, London.

Nazroo J Y (1997a) *The Health of Britain's Ethnic Minorities*. Policy Studies Institute, London.

Nazroo J Y (1997b) *Ethnicity and Mental Health: Findings from a National Community Survey*. Policy Studies Institute, London.

Nazroo J Y (1997c) Health and health services. In Modood T, Berthoud R, Lakey J, Smith P, Virdee S and Beishon S (1997) *Ethnic Minorities in Britain: Diversity and Disadvantage*. Policy Studies Institute, London, pp. 224–58.

Nazroo J Y (1998) Genetic, cultural or socio-economic vulnerability? Explaining ethnic inequalities in health. *Sociology of Health and Illness* **20**(5): 710–30.

NHS Confederation (1998) *Composite Directory of NHS Ethnic Health Unit Projects*. The NHS Confederation, Birmingham.

NHS Development Unit (1998) *Supporting Guidance to HSC 1998/139: Developing Primary Care Groups*. Department of Health, Leeds.

NHS Executive (1992) *Local Voices: The Views of Local People in Purchasing for Health*. Department of Health, London.

NHS Executive (1994) *Collection of Ethnic Group Data for Admitted Patients*. EL(94)77. NHS Executive, Leeds.

NHS Executive (1995) *The Patient's Charter and You*. Department of Health, London.

NHS Management Executive (1993) *Ethnic Minority Staff in the NHS: A Programme of Action*. EL(94)12. Department of Health, London.

Norman A (1985) *Triple Jeopardy: Growing Old in a Second Homeland*. Policy Studies in Ageing No. 3. Centre for Policy on Ageing, London.

Nuffield Council on Bioethics (1993) *Genetic Screening: Ethical Issues*. Nuffield Foundation, London.

Nurses, Midwives and Health Visitors Rules Approval Order 1983, Statutory Instrument No. 873. HMSO, London.

O'Donnell O and Popper C (1991) Equity and distribution of NHS resources. *Journal of Health Economics* **10**: 1–19.

Office of Population Censuses and Surveys/Office for National Statistics (1994) *Undercoverage in Great Britain* (Census User Guide no. 58). HMSO, London.

Ostrowsky J, Lippman A and Scriver C (1985) Cost-benefit analysis of a thalassaemia disease prevention program. *American Journal of Public Health* **75**(7): 732–6.

Parkin F (1979) *Marxism and Class Theory: A Bourgeois Critique.* Tavistock, London.

Parsons L and Day S (1992) Improving obstetric outcomes in ethnic minorities: an evaluation of health advocacy in Hackney. *Journal of Public Health Medicine* **14**(2): 183–91.

Parsons T (1951) *The Social System.* Free Press, New York.

Patterson S (1965) *Dark Strangers: A Study of West Indians in London.* Penguin, Harmondsworth.

Peach C (1986) *West Indian Migration to Britain.* Oxford University Press, Oxford.

Peach C (1991) *The Caribbean in Europe: contrasting patterns of migration and settlement.* Centre for Research in Ethnic Relations, Coventry.

Peach C (ed) (1996a) *Ethnicity in the Census Volume 2.* HMSO, London.

Peach C (1996b) Introduction. In Peach C (ed) *Ethnicity in the Census Volume 2.* HMSO, London, pp. 1–24.

Pearson M (1986a) Racist notions of ethnicity and culture in health education. In Rodmell S and Watt A (1986) *The Politics of Health Education.* Routledge and Kegan Paul, London, pp. 38–56.

Pearson M (1986b) The politics of ethnic minority health studies. In Rathwell T and Phillips D (eds) *Health, Race and Ethnicity.* Croom Helm, London, pp. 100–16.

Perry S I, Shu R T, Brooks W and Cherry D (1999) Perceptions of community services among Asian and White stroke survivors and their carers: an exploratory study *Ethnicity and Health* **4**(1/2): 101–5.

Pharoah C (1995) *Primary Health Care for Elderly People from Black and Minority Ethnic Communities.* Studies in Ageing. Age Concern/Institute of Gerontology, King's College. HMSO, London.

Phelan M and Parkman S (1995) Work with an interpreter. *British Medical Journal* **311**: 555–7.

Phillips M and Phillips T (1998) *Windrush: The Irresistible Rise of Multi-Racial Britain.* Harper Collins, London.

Phizacklea A (1984) A sociology of migration or 'race relations'? *Current Sociology* **32**(4): 199–218.

Phizacklea A and Miles R (1992) The British trade union movement and racism. In Braham P, Rattansi A and Skellington E (eds) *Racism and Antiracism: Inequalities, Opportunities and Policies.* Sage, London, pp. 30–45.

Phoenix A (1991) *Young Mothers?* Polity Press, London.

Pointon T (1996) Telephone interpreting service is available. *British Medical Journal* **312**: 53.

Porter R (1991) 'Expressing yourself ill': the language of sickness in Georgian England. In Burke P and Porter R *Language, self and society: a social history of language.* Polity Press, Cambridge, pp. 276–99.

Porter S (1992) The poverty of professionalization: a critical analysis of strategies for the occupational advancement of nursing. *Journal of Advanced Nursing* **17**: 720–6.

Porter S (1993) Critical realist ethnography: the case of racism and professionalism in a medical setting. *Sociology* **27**(4): 591–609.

Porter S (1998) *Social Theory and Nursing Practice.* Macmillan, Basingstoke.

Pringle M and Rothera I (1996) Practicality of recording patient ethnicity in general practice *British Medical Journal* **107**: 1080–82.

Pringle M, Rothera I, McNichol K and Boot D (1997) *Ethnic Group Data Collection in Primary Care.* University of Nottingham, Department of General Practice, Monograph 3, Nottingham.

Pudney S and Shields M (1997) *Gender and Racial Equality in Pay and Promotion in the Internal Labour Market for NHS Nurses.* Centre for Public Sector Economic Research, University of Leicester.

Quill T E (1989) Recognizing and adjusting to barriers in doctor-patient communication. *Annals of Internal Medicine* **111**: 51–7.

Qureshi B (1989) *Transcultural Medicine.* Kluwer Academic, Dordrecht.

Rack P (1990) Psychological/psychiatric disorders. In McAvoy B R and Donaldson L J (eds) *Health Care for Asians.* Routledge, London, pp. 290–303.

Rader G S (1988) Management decisions: do we really need interpreters? *Nursing Management* **19**(7): 46–8.

Raleigh V S (1996) Suicide patterns and trends in people of Indian subcontinent and Caribbean origin in England and Wales. *Ethnicity and Health* **1**(1): 55–63.

Raleigh V S, Bulusu L and Balarajan R (1990) Suicides among immigrants from the Indian subcontinent. *British Journal of Psychiatry* **156**: 46–50.

Raleigh V S and Balarajan R (1992) Suicide and self-burning among Indians and West Indians in England and Wales. *British Journal of Psychiatry* **161**: 365–8.

Raleigh V S, Kiri V and Balarajan R (1997) Variations in mortality from diabetes mellitus, hypertension and renal disease in England and Wales by country of birth. *Health Trends* **28**(4): 122–7.

Ramdin R (1987) *The Making of the Black Working Class in Britain.* Gower, Aldershot.

Rampton B (1995) *Crossing: Language and Ethnicity Among Adolescents.* Longman, Harlow.

Ranger C (1994) King's Evidence. *Health Service Journal* **104**: 22–3.

Ratip S, Skuse D, Porter J, Wonke B, Yardumian A and Modell B (1995) Psychological and clinical burden of thalassaemia intermedia and its implications for prenatal diagnosis. *Archives of Disease in Childhood* **72**: 408–12.

Rattansi A (1992) Changing the Subject? Racism, culture and education. In Donald J and Rattansi A (eds) *'Race', Culture and Difference.* Sage, London, pp. 11–48.

Rattansi A (1994) Western racisms, ethnicities and identities in a 'postmodern' frame. In Rattansi A and Westwood S (eds) *Racism, Modernity and Identity on the Western Front.* Polity Press, Cambridge, pp. 15–86.

Ravaioli M (1997) UFOL: unidentified fragments of language. The English review of papers of medical and scientific research. *Journal of Experimental and Clinical Cancer Research* **16**(2): 233–4.

Reeves F (1989) *Race and Borough Politics.* Research in Ethnic Relations Series. Avebury, Aldershot.

Rehman R and Walker E (1995) Researching black and minority ethnic groups. *Health Education Journal* **54**: 489–500.

Rex J (1970) *Race Relations and Sociological Theory.* Routledge and Kegan Paul, London.

Rex J (1986) *Race and Ethnicity.* Open University Press, Milton Keynes.

Rhodes P (1994) Race-of-Interviewer Effects: a brief comment. *Sociology* **28**(2): 547–58.

Rocheron Y (1991) The Asian Mother and Baby Campaign: the construction of ethnic minorities' health needs. In Loney M, Bocock R, Clarke J, Cochrane A, Graham P and Wilson M (eds) *The State or the Market: Politics and Welfare in Contemporary Britain.* Sage, London, pp. 184–205.

Rogers A (1990) Policing mental disorder: controversies, myths and realities. *Social Policy and Administration* **24**(3): 226–36.

Rogers R (1992) Living and dying in the USA: sociodemographic determinants of death among blacks and whites. *Demography* **29**(2): 287–303.

Rose S (1997) *Lifelines: Biology, Determinism and Freedom.* Penguin/Allen Lane, Harmondsworth.

Rose S, Lewontin R and Kamin L (1984) *Not In Our Genes: Biology, Ideology and Human Nature.* Penguin, Harmondsworth.

Rose S and Rose H (1986) Less than human nature. *Race and Class* **27**(3): 47–66.

Rothman B K (1994) *The Tentative Pregnancy* (revised edn). Pandora, London

Rudat K (1994) *Black and Ethnic Minority Groups in England: Health and Lifestyles.* Health Education Authority, London.

Sainsburys Centre for Mental Health (1998a) *Keys to Engagement: Review of Care For People With Severe Mental Illness Who Are Hard to Engage With Services.* Sainsburys Centre for Mental Health, London.

Sainsburys Centre for Mental Health (1998b) *Acute Problems: A Survey of the Quality of Care in Acute Psychiatric Wards.* Sainsburys Centre for Mental Health, London.

Salter B (1998) *The Politics of Change in the Health Service.* Macmillan Press – now Palgrave, Basingstoke.

Salvage J (1985) *The Politics of Nursing.* Heinemann Nursing, Oxford.

Sashidharan S P (1993) Afro-Caribbeans and schizophrenia: the ethnic vulnerability hypothesis re-examined. *International Review of Psychiatry* **5**: 129–44.

Sashidharan S and Francis E (1993) Epidemiology, ethnicity and schizophrenia. In Ahmad, W I U (ed) *'Race' and Health in Contemporary Britain.* Open University Press, Buckingham.

Schaeffer N C (1980) Evaluating race-of-interviewer effects in a national survey. *Sociological Methods and Research* **8**(4): 400–19.

Schott J and Henley A (1996) *Culture, Religion and Childbearing in a Multiracial Society: A Handbook for Health Professionals.* Butterworth-Heinemann, Oxford.

Schulte R (1996) Editorial: a blueprint for translation studies. *Translation Review* **51, 52**: 1–4.

Schuman H and Converse J M (1971) The effects of black and white interviewers on black responses in 1968. *Public Opinion Quarterly* **35**: 48–68.

Scruton R (1986) The myth of cultural relativism. In Palmer F (ed) *Anti-Racism – an Assault on Education and Value.* Sherwood Press, London: pp. 127–35.

Sheldon T and Parker H (1992) Race and ethnicity in health research. *Journal of Public Health Medicine* **14**(2): 104–10.

Silverman D (1993) *Interpreting Qualitative Data: methods for analysing text, talk and interaction.* Sage, London.

Smaje C (1995a) *Health, 'Race' and Ethnicity: Making Sense of the Evidence.* King's Fund, London.

Smaje C (1995b) Ethnic residential concentration and health: evidence for a beneficial effect? *Policy and Politics* **23**(3): 251–69.

Smaje C (1996) The ethnic patterning of health: new directions for theory and research. *Sociology of Health and Illness* **18**(2): 139–71.

Smaje C (1997) Not just a social construct: theorising race and ethnicity. *Sociology* **31**(2): 307–27.

Smaje C and Field D (1997) Absent minorities? Ethnicity and the use of palliative care services. In Field D, Hockey J and Small N (eds) *Death, Gender and Ethnicity.* Routledge, London, pp. 166–86.

Smaje C and Le Grand J (1997) Ethnicity, equity and the use of health services in the British NHS. *Social Science and Medicine* **45**: 485–96.

Small S (1994) Black people in Britain. *Sociology Review* **3**(4): 2–4.

Smart B (1983) *Foucault, Marxism and Critique.* Routledge and Kegan Paul, London.

Smith D J (1980) *Overseas Doctors in the National Health Service.* Policy Studies Institute, London.

Smith D K, Slack J and Shaw R W *et al.* (1994) Lack of knowledge in health professionals: a barrier to providing information to patients? *Quality in Health Care* **3**: 75–8.

Smith J and Pankhania G (1996) *Cultural Awareness Resource Pack.* Public Relations Division, North West Anglia Health Authority, Peterborough.

Smith J A, Epseland M, Bellevue R, Bonds D, Brown A K and Koshy M (1996) Pregnancy in sickle cell disease: experience of the co-operative study of sickle cell disease. *Obstetrics and Gynaecology* **87**(2): 199–204.

Snell J (1997) Joke Over. *Nursing Times* **93**(11): 26–9.

Sokoloff N J (1992) *Black Women and White Women in the Professions.* Routledge, London.

Solomos J and Back L (1996) *Racism and Society.* Macmillan, London.

Sondhi R (1987) *Divided Families: British Immigration Control in the Indian Sub-Continent.* Runnymede Trust, London.

Stolk Y, Ziguras S, Saunders T, Garlick R, Stuart G and Coffey G (1998) Lowering the language barrier in an acute psychiatric setting. *Australian and New Zealand Journal of Psychiatry* **32**: 434–40.

Stone D H and Stewart S (1996) Screening and the new genetics; a public health perspective on the ethical debate. *Journal of Public Health Medicine* **18**(1): 3–5.

Stuart G W, Minas I H, Klimidis S and O'Connell S (1996) English language ability and mental health service utilisation: a census. *Australian and New Zealand Journal of Psychiatry* **30**: 270–77.

Stubbs P (1993) 'Ethnically sensitive' or 'anti-racist'? models for health research and service delivery. In Ahmad W I U (ed) *'Race' and Health in Contemporary Britain.* Open University Press, Buckingham, pp. 34–50.

Sue D W (1994) (7th edn) A model for cultural diversity training. In Samovar L and Porter R (eds) *Inter-cultural Communication: a Reader.* Wadsworth, Belmont, California.

Swarup N (1993) *Equal Voice: Black Communities' Views on Housing, Health and Social Services.* Report No. 22. Social Services Research and Information Unit, Portsmouth Polytechnic, Portsmouth.

Sweeting H and West P (1995) Family life and health in adolescence: a role for culture in the health inequalities debate. *Social Science and Medicine* **40**(2): 163–75.

Takei N, Persaud R, Woodruff P, Brockington I and Murray R M (1998) First episodes of psychosis in Afro-Caribbean and White people. *British Journal of Psychiatry* **172**: 147–53.

Thomas M and Morton-Williams J (1972) *Overseas Nurses in Britain: A PEP Survey for the UK.* Council Broadsheet no. 539. Political and Economic Planning (now Policy Studies Institute), London.

Thomas V and Dines A (1994) The health needs of ethnic minority groups: are nurses and individuals playing their part? *Journal of Advanced Nursing* **20**: 802–8.

Thomasma D C (1994) Models of the doctor-patient relationship and the ethics committee: part two. *Cambridge Quarterly of Healthcare Ethics* **3**: 10–26.

Torres R E (1998) The pervading role of language on health. *Journal of Health Care for the Poor and Underserved* **9** (supplement): 18–19.

Totten V Y, Knopp R, Helpern K, Hauswald M, Vicellio P, Brennan J, Rosenzweig S and Jesionek P (1996) Physician-patient communication in the emergency department. Part 2: communication strategies for specific situations. *Academic Emergency Medicine* **3**(12): 1146–53.

Townsend P (1979) *Poverty in the United Kingdom. A survey of household resources and standards of living.* Penguin, Harmondsworth.

Townsend P, Davidson N and Whitehead M (1988) *Inequalities in health. The Black Report and the Health Divide.* Penguin, Harmondsworth.

Tuffnell D, Nuttall K, Raistrick J and Jackson T (1994) Use of translated written material to communicate with non-English speaking patients. *British Medical Journal* **309**: 992.

Twigg J and Atkin K (1994) *Carers Perceived: Policy and Practice in Informal Care.* Open University Press, Buckingham.

UKCC (1989) UKCC requirements for the content of Project 2000 programmes. PS&D/89/04 (B). UKCC, London.

UKCC (April 1998) *Standards for specialist education and practice.* UKCC, London.

U.K. Thalassaemia Society (1988) *Do you, your parents, or your grandparents come from . . . ?* (Poster) U.K. Thalassaemia Society, London.

Vandenbroucke J P, van der Meer F J M, Helmerhorst F M and Rosendaal, F R (1996) Factor V Leiden: should we screen oral contraceptive users and pregnant women? *British Medical Journal* **313**: 1127–30.

Van Os J, Castle D J, Takei N, Der G and Murray R M (1996) Psychotic illness in ethnic minorities: clarification from the 1991 Census. *Psychological Medicine* **26**: 203–8.

Venuti L (1995) *The translator's invisibility: a history of translation.* Routledge, London.

Vermeulen H (ed) (1997) *Immigration Policy for a Multi-cultural Society.* Migration Policy Group, Brussels.

Virdee S (1995) *Racial Violence and Harassment.* Policy Studies Institute, London.

Virdee S (1997) Racial Harassment. In Modood T, Berthoud R, Lakey J, Nazroo J, Smith P, Virdee S and Beishon S (eds) *Ethnic Minorities in Britain: Diversity and Disadvantage.* Policy Studies Institute, London.

Vu H H-T (1996) Cultural barriers between obstetrician-gynecologists and Vietnamese/Chinese immigrant women. *Texas Medicine* **92**(10): 47–52.

Waddell C and McNamara B (1997) The stereotypical fallacy: a comparison of Anglo and Chinese Australians' thoughts about facing death. *Mortality* **2**(2): 149–61.

Wallman S (ed) (1979) *Ethnicity at Work.* Macmillan, London.

Wallman S (1986) Ethnicity and the boundary process in context. In Rex J and Mason D (eds) *Theories of Race and Ethnic Relations.* Cambridge University Press, Cambridge, pp. 226–45.

Ward L (1993) Race equality and employment in the National Health Service. In Ahmad W I U (ed) *'Race' and Health in Contemporary Britain*. Open University Press, Buckingham, pp. 167–82.

Ward-Collins D (1998) 'Noncompliant.' Isn't there a better way to say it? *American Journal of Nursing* **98**(5): 27–31.

Wardhaugh R (1986) *An Introduction to Sociolinguistics*. Blackwell, Oxford.

Wardhaugh R (1987) *Languages in competition: dominance, diversity and decline*. Blackwell, Oxford.

Webbe A (1998) Ethnicity and Mental Health. *Psychiatric Care* **5**(1): 12–16.

Wedderburn Tate C (1996) Race into action. *Nursing Times* **92**(22): 28–30.

Wedderburn Tate C (1998) Ethnic Lessons, *Nursing Management* **5**(1): 5.

Wessel L A (1998) Translation Trouble. *The Nurse Practitioner* June: 11.

White M and Epston D (1990) *Narrative Means to Therapeutic Ends*. W W Norton, New York.

Whyte W F (1984) *Learning from the Field*. Sage, London.

Wilkinson G and Miers M (1999) *Power and Nursing Practice*. Macmillan, Basingstoke.

Wilkinson J (1998) Non-compliance by patients: a response to Professor Dimond. *Nursing Ethics* **5**(2): 167–72.

Wilkinson R G (1996) *Unhealthy Societies: The Afflictions of Inequality*. Routledge, London.

Wilkinson S and Kitzinger C (1996) *Representing The Other: A Feminism and Psychology Reader*. Sage, London.

Williams D, Takeuchi D and Adair R (1992) Marital status and psychiatric disorder among blacks and whites. *Journal of Health and Social Behaviour* **33**: 140–57.

Williams R (1993) Health and length of residence among South Asians in Glasgow: a study controlling for age. *Journal of Public Health Medicine* **15**(1): 52–60.

Williams R, Eley S, Hunt K and Bhatt S (1997) Has psychological distress among UK South Asians been underestimated? A comparison of three measures in the west of Scotland population. *Ethnicity and Health* **2**(1/2): 21–9.

Wilson D A (1989) My trips over the language barrier. *American Journal of Nursing* December: 1718.

Witz A (1992) *Professions and Patriarchy*. Routledge, London.

Woloshin S, Schwartz L M, Katz S J and Welch H G (1997) Is language a barrier to the use of preventive services? *Journal of General Internal Medicine* **12**(8): 472–7.

World Health Organization (1988) *The Haemoglobinopathies in Europe: combined report of two WHO meetings* (Document EUR/ICP/MCH 110). WHO Regional Office for Europe, Copenhagen.

World Health Organization (1992) *International Classification of Mental and Behavioural Disorders*. World Health Organization, Geneva.

World Health Organization (1993) *Health for all targets. The health policy for Europe.* European Health for All Series No 4. WHO Regional Office for Europe, Copenhagen.

World Health Organization (1994) *Guidelines for the control of haemoglobin disorders.* Unpublished WHO document of the WHO working group on haemoglobinopathies, Cagliari, Sardinia 8–9 April 1989. World Health Organization, Geneva.

Wright C M (1994) Language and communication problems in an Asian community. *Journal of the Royal College of General Practitioners* **33**: 101–4.

Young P (1999) Tales from little India. Southall Black Sisters. BBC, Radio 4, 31 March.

Zeuner D, Ades A E, Karnon J, Brown J, Dezateux C and Anionwu E N (1999) Antenatal and neonatal haemoglobinopathy screening in the UK: review and economic analysis. *Health Technology Assessment* **3**(11).

Index of names

Subject index